Pathways to Pain Relief

Frances Sommer Anderson, PhD, SEP
Eric Sherman, PsyD

For
John E. Sarno, MD
&
Our Patients

Pathways to Pain Relief is based upon the pioneering work of John E. Sarno, MD, Professor of Rehabilitation Medicine, New York University School of Medicine. Dr. Sarno has advanced the idea that a wide variety of pain disorders are psychophysiologic in origin. Psychophysiologic disorders, previously referred to as psychosomatic disorders, are just one aspect of the recently energized field of mindbody medicine.

What distinguishes *Pathways to Pain Relief* is that it embraces the position that musculoskeletal pain and other psychophysiologic disorders can originate from psychological experiences as a means to protect an individual from unbearable emotional distress. Psychotherapeutic techniques based on the medicalization of musculoskeletal pain foreclose the possibility of approaching these conditions as a psychophysiologic disorder. The medicalization paradigm prevents many clinicians from recognizing that the same emotional conflicts which lead to psychological symptoms can initiate the development of physical symptoms as well. *Pathways to Pain Relief* provides details on how treatment has worked from the patient's and the therapist's point of view. The authors, Dr. Frances Sommer Anderson & Dr. Eric Sherman, present clinical case material to illustrate how musculoskeletal pain and other psychophysiologic disorders can originate from psychological experiences as a means to protect an individual from unbearable emotional distress.

Copyright © 2013 Frances Sommer Anderson & Eric Sherman

ISBN: 1484016718

ISBN-13: 978-1484016718

Book Design by Sergio Quiros: sergioquiros@me.com

Cover artwork photography: *Texture of Time*, 2003 by Frances Sommer Anderson

CONTENTS

Acknowledgments	xiii
Foreword: John E. Sarno, MD	xxi
Frances Sommer Anderson, PhD, SEP Introduction	1
Defining Pain	3
Treating Tension Myoneural Syndrome—(TMS)	6
References	15
Eric Sherman, PsyD Introduction	17
Defining TMS	18
(Mis)Diagnosing TMS	22
TMS: An Historical Perspective	24
The (Mis)Treatment of Pain Symptomatology	26
Technical Considerations	28

Disconnecting and Reconnecting with Feelings	34
Clinical Implications: Two Case Histories	40
Critiques of Dr. Sarno's Contributions	51
Summary	52
Pain Vignettes	57
Perfectionism and Goodism	58
Personality Development and Cognitive Development	64
Anger and Self-Sacrifice	76
The Lethality of Anger	82
Childhood Experience	85
Experiencing the Past in a New Way	89
The Reawakening of Childhood Trauma	94
TMS as Adaptation to Stress	102
External Stressors vs. Childhood Experience	105
References	109

Frances Sommer Anderson, PhD, SEP 113
TREATING TMS PAIN: ILLUSTRATING
THE CLINICAL PROCESS

Becoming Aware of and Learning to Tolerate 115
Overwhelming Emotions Relieves TMS Pain
Ellen's Story

Overwhelming Experiences in Childhood and 139
Adulthood
Sessions with Mrs. R

Little Kate's Journey 156

The Legacy of Harsh Parenting 164
Mr. L and The Tenacious Inner Critic

Self-Sufficient, Too Early 168
Ms. T

Speaking Up for Myself 180
Mr. A

Discussion 188

CONCLUSION 195
Eric Sherman & Frances Sommer Anderson

About the Authors 200

Acknowledgments

Learning to help people find relief from pain has been the focus of my clinical practice since 1979, when I was a member of the Psychology Department at Rusk Institute-NYU Langone Medical Center. Arlene Feinblatt, PhD, the psychologist who worked with John E. Sarno, MD in developing his approach to treating Tension Myoneural Syndrome (TMS) pain, invited me to join her in working with Dr. Sarno's patients. I am eternally grateful to her for the opportunity of a lifetime—to learn from her and Dr. Sarno, pioneers in the field of mindbody medicine. Collaborating with the rehabilitation team to help people with the most challenging, intractable pain syndromes changed the course of my career, stimulating my search for knowledge and skills in the domain of psychoanalysis.

Discoveries during my treatment of Ellen, one of Dr. Sarno's patients, had such an impact that I wrote a psychoanalytic paper about our work together, published in 1998 in *Relational Perspectives on the Body*, co-edited with Lewis Aron. Lew's invitation to co-edit the book, now a foundational psychoanalytic text, heralded a recognition of the need to bring the "body" back into the world of psychoanalysis. Lew Aron has continued to be a generative mentor, fostering creativity and steadfastly supporting my attempts to move deeper into unexplored mindbody territory, reflected in my edited book, *Bodies in Treatment: The Unspoken Dimension*, published in 2008.

When I developed chronic tension-related headaches in 1983, I was impelled to search for relief, broadly and deeply in my personal psychoanalysis. My experience of being in pain and finding relief through psychotherapeutic intervention has enhanced my ability to help others find relief. Discovering residues of prenatal, perinatal, and postnatal emotional trauma, in addition to attachment trauma in the first two years of my life, has propelled me into intensive study of the neurobiology of pain, trauma, and attachment. Thus, helping people in pain is a personal and professional quest, still in progress.

In 1987, I left Rusk Institute for full-time private practice and psychoanalytic training. I continued to collaborate with Dr. Sarno in treating his patients, through his retirement from medical practice in April 2012, and beyond, staying in touch for infusions of inspiration, wisdom, and humor. Thank you, Dr. Sarno, and Martha Taylor Sarno, for trusting me in a substantive, mutative professional undertaking…and for friendship that endures. Thank you, Mary Oland, Dr. Sarno's office manager, who manifested grace under pressure, enabling each of us to be optimally responsive and responsible.

While at Rusk, I met my co-author, Eric Sherman, PsyD. In 1983, he worked as a clinical psychology intern under Dr. Feinblatt's supervision on Dr. Sarno's Pain Service. As Co-Director of the Clinical Psychology Internship Program at Rusk, I also taught and supervised Dr. Sherman. His facility for treating people in pain was quickly apparent. When Dr. Sherman joined the Psychology Department Staff at Rusk, we became colleagues, benefitting mutually from consulting about our clinical challenges. Our psychoanalytic training at the New York University Postdoctoral Program in Psychotherapy and

Psychoanalysis overlapped: We graduated together in 1999. I invited him to co-author this book of case studies in treating Dr. Sarno's patients, knowing that our clinical competencies would complement the project, enriching it because of our distinctive skills and approaches to writing about our work. Further, I knew that we share a passion for communicating what we have learned to a wide readership, aiming to offer our many years of clinical wisdom directly to people in pain.

Shortly after we forged our pledge to write this volume, we had the opportunity to participate in founding a non-profit educational corporation, the Psychophysiologic Disorders Association (PPDA), dedicated to expanding discoveries about musculoskeletal pain as a mindbody disorder and extending the reach of medical and psychological intervention to other mindbody conditions. Although delaying the publication of *Pathways to Pain Relief*, we were committed to advancing the mission of the PPDA. We co-chaired "When Stress Causes Pain: Innovative Treatments for Psychophysiologic Disorders," a national conference held at the New York Academy of Medicine in New York City, October 6, 2012. I am grateful for the two years of committed focus of all of the members of the Planning Committee for the conference: It was a transforming experience. Attended by 250 participants, the conference was co-sponsored by the Psychophysiologic Disorders Association and the New York University Postdoctoral Program in Psychotherapy and Psychoanalysis, a ground-breaking collaboration between medical practitioners, mental health clinicians, and health care consumer advocates.

Along this path, I have been sustained and stimulated by my psychoanalysts, teachers, publishers, colleagues, bodyworkers, and friends too numerous to name here. If you are reading this, I acknowledge you with boundless gratitude and respect.

To my patients, thank you for teaching me, inspiring me with your courage, and trusting me to enter most closely guarded interiors in order for us to relieve your somatic and emotional pain. To those I have not been able to help as much as we had hoped was possible, I hope that you have found relief with the help of others.

Thank you, Eric, for helping me navigate personal and professional tsunamis. You have modeled being the flexible palm tree that can survive assaults from all directions.

Sergio Quiros, your technical and esthetic assistance in designing this book took this project from fermentation as a Word document revised countless times to digital publication. Thank you for your patience and tolerance of our demands and for urging us to press on and reach a higher level of creativity.

While this endeavor was in progress, my husband, William Sommer, died suddenly. Bill, thank you for being another stalwart palm tree from the beginning of my quest to help people find relief from pain. You believed in me, fully supported my dedication to my patients, and tolerated, usually with equanimity, the long hours I devoted to my professional development.

Thank you to several generations of feline comforters, Yitzak, Herzog, Fog, Sweetie, and Lovey. You have taught me most of what I know about nonverbal communication.

FSA

To Dr. John E. Sarno and my patients, whose generosity, wisdom, and courage have taught, inspired, and enabled me to help people suffering from psychophysiologic disorders.

To Dr. Arlene Feinblatt, "the Mother of All TMS Therapists" and my first teacher, whose patience and belief in me were gifts that still touch me.

To Dr. Donnel Stern, who helped me find my own path to write this book. To my friend, colleague, and co-author, Dr. Frances S. Anderson, who has been both the midwife and shepherd to me throughout the entire process of developing, writing, and publishing this book.

To Mary Oland, Dr. Sarno's long-time secretary, who is the operational definition of grace under pressure.

To Sergio Quiros, a true renaissance man, whose invaluable assistance on this book and other related projects has enabled me to have a life.

And to my husband, Michael McCabe, I couldn't possibly thank him enough for all his support and encouragement during this project and always.

ES

FOREWORD

As one views the contemporary medical scene in the United States, it is apparent that the specialty of mindbody medicine does not exist in this country. Because of the widely held pejorative connotations of the word psychosomatic, I have chosen not to use it, though it should be clearly understood that the words *mindbody* and *psychosomatic* are synonymous.

The practice of mindbody medicine mandates a liaison between a physician and a psychologist trained to understand the psychodynamics involved in mindbody disorders (for the purposes of this piece, the term *psychologist* will include psychiatrists). The reason for the partnership is based on the fact that only a physician can evaluate symptomatology and determine whether it is the result of a disease or a mindbody disorder. The role of the psychologist is obvious. There, however, is the rub, for today's physicians are constitutionally incapable of attributing any symptom to a mindbody process, so all medical ills are "organic," meaning it's all in the body and has nothing to do with the mind. That medical failure is the basis for the pain epidemic (mostly back) that has been in existence for many years. Is it liable to change? Not as long as the epidemic continues to be a medical cash cow, and it is, with more entering the cattle business every day. Now, neuroscientists are offering to cure chronic back pain with an incredible machine that will show you exactly what your brain is doing (*New York Times*, August 26, 2007).

So much for the grim, sardonic, tragic situation that characterizes American medicine today. The authors of this book tell the stories of a group of people who survived conventional medical mismanagement, were properly diagnosed, engaged in a psychoeducational program under my tutelage, and completed their treatment with the authors.

The proper diagnosis is a mindbody disorder in which people may experience pain, a variety of sensations called paresthesias (numbness, tingling, burning, etc.) and muscle weakness in the trunk, legs, and arms. Symptoms are highly individual. Of these, pain is the most consistent and disabling and the one for which most people seek treatment.

The pathophysiology—that is, the actual physical process that is responsible for the symptoms—is rather straightforward. What one might refer to as the unconscious decision-maker in the brain/mind concludes that the emotional situation has reached a critical point and that something must be done to reinforce the normal forces of repression, the process that is designed to keep dangerous, painful, unhappy, embarrassing, or otherwise unacceptable emotions locked up in the unconscious. It is a decision made without consulting the conscious decision-maker, which seems illogical but which is the reality of brain function at this point in evolutionary time. I shall discuss later the basis for the decision, but its physical result is to render targeted anatomical structures mildly oxygen-deprived, which is the immediate cause of the symptoms. Fortunately, it is a benign process; that is, no damage is done to the targeted tissues, though they are rendered "dysfunctional," which is the basis for symptoms. As stated above, these symptoms are invariably attributed to a host of structural abnormalities, almost all of which are the result of aging, and not pathological. My books have described this process in detail. I call the disorder the Tension Myoneural Syndrome (TMS).

Now to the heart of the matter, which is not at all straightforward: the psychology behind the physical manifestations. What follows is the result of work with thousands of patients over almost four decades, a lot of reading in psychology and discussion with the psychologists who work with me. I am prepared to alter the ideas to be set forth at any time, as long as it is acknowledged that their origin is psychosomatic.

Long before the details of the psychodynamic became evident, it seemed clear that some unconscious process was at work. Eventually, it was concluded that symptoms were created to reinforce repression by mounting a physical distraction, and that the severity of the symptoms reflected the intensity of the emotional state that required them. In other words, the symptoms were designed to protect the individual from the conscious experience of strong emotions. The obvious questions: What are those emotions, and what is their genesis?

At first glance, it is hard to believe that the most important feeling is unconscious rage. The idea is threatening, preposterous, frightening to most people, but there is reason to believe that, with variations, unconscious rage is universal, part of the human condition in our culture at this point in evolutionary time. Consideration of its sources will make the idea more acceptable. As will be seen, it is not the only unconscious feeling that contributes to the necessity for symptoms, but is clearly the most powerful. It must be noted, however, that the rage is only a brief step away from the symptom designed to repress it, separated only by the "wall" that separates the conscious and unconscious spheres of mental-emotional activity. Experience has taught us that trying to express this unconscious rage is fruitless, though patients invariably ask how to do it. We have found, on the other hand, that becoming aware of the feelings that give rise to the rage can have a strong therapeutic effect.

It should come as no surprise that the first contributor to the reservoir of rage we accumulate as we go through life is childhood. In fact, the influence of childhood emotional experiences is probably responsible for the majority of the rage, as will be seen as we go along. In the first five or six years of life, we are primarily emotional beings. It would, therefore, be logical that whatever reactions we have will be unrelated to reason or thought. It is essential, therefore, that the predominant feeling to be conveyed to the child be unconditional love and acceptance. Historically, this has rarely been the case. Outright physical, sexual, or emotional abuse will give rise to monumental pain, hurt, sadness, and anger, all repressed, for children are protected from such feelings by the mind. I have found, however, that what might be called subtle emotional abuse is virtually universal in previous generations. It was my personal experience. Instead of unconditional love and total acceptance, we learned to conduct ourselves within behavioral parameters set forth by our parents, either explicitly or by implication. Examples: One must be good all the time; anger is not allowed; one must please mommy and daddy; children should be seen and not heard; you'd better be good or I will tell your father; the constant threat of punishment. In the years that follow, after some teenage revolt, we become compliant adults, who need to prove ourselves all the time by performing perfectly and by being "very good people.". I have dubbed these tendencies "the perfect and the good." They are universal in the people I have worked with over the years. Without realizing it, we live our lives conforming to what we think is expected of us. This has very little to do with achievements, success in careers, and the like, but it has everything to do with our personal lives and how we feel as we go through life.

Of necessity, this is a brief discussion of an important, potentially complicated subject. The combination of unconscious anger generated during the early childhood years and that which accumulates throughout life due to the pressures we put on ourselves to be perfect and good account for most of the reservoir of rage, hurt, sadness, and fear that are the legacy of childhood. The last contributors to the rage reservoir are the stressful things that happen to us as we go through life. Since these are the only pressures we are aware of, it is natural to conclude that they are the sole reason for the imposition of physical symptoms when, in fact, they are only the last straw (more appropriately, the last brick).

The therapeutic approach to relieving the person's pain has been developed over the years by trial and error, though it was realized fairly early in the game that teaching the sufferer what was going on both physically and psychologically, and how they were related, seemed to be of great value. It was a pleasant surprise to learn that reading even the first book, published in 1984, "cured" some people, though it lacked any discussion of the psychological process described above. This was a clear demonstration of the therapeutic power of information. Succeeding books have done the same thing. Increasing knowledge of the nature of TMS, and greater sophistication in the presentation of the information, have contributed to success in dealing with the disorder.

In about one quarter of our patients, psychotherapy is essential for success. These patients harbor feelings that are deeply repressed in the unconscious and can only be brought to consciousness with the help of appropriately trained psychotherapists. The authors of this book have had years of experience working with TMS, and bring to their interaction with the patient not only their knowledge of TMS, but also great sensitivity and insight into the mysterious ways of the human unconscious. They have been of crucial importance in the lives of many of our patients. The case histories in this book are illustrative of their successful management of people with severe TMS.

John E. Sarno, MD
January 2010

Frances Sommer Anderson

Introduction[1]

Pamela, 36, a physically-fit, accomplished professional woman juggling career and two children under age 4, is sitting at the holiday dinner table in her home, listening to her adored and adoring father regale the family with anecdotes from childhood about her and her brother, 2 years younger. He turns to her and says, "Oh, Pamela, you know you were never good in math and geography." Only a few minutes later, she feels sharp pain in her back. The pain is so severe that she excuses herself and goes into her kitchen to calm her reaction to the pain and to identify the emotional trigger for its sudden onset.

Using the work we have done in psychoanalytic psychotherapy for the past year, she quickly realizes that she is furious at her father for his "sexist" point of view.

How could he say that, knowing so well her passionate feminist leanings? Within a few minutes, the pain vanishes and she's able to return to the dining table.

This is one of numerous, dramatic examples of the relationship between bodily pain and emotions that my co-author, Eric Sherman, PsyD, and I have witnessed since 1979 while treating people diagnosed with Tension Myoneural Syndrome (TMS) by John E. Sarno, MD, Professor of Rehabilitation Medicine at Rusk Institute-New York University Langone Medical Center. As he elaborated in his four books and in peer-reviewed journal articles, TMS is mediated by feelings, or emotions, that are so unacceptable, so threatening (e.g., anger, fear, shame, guilt, or even love), that they cannot be experienced consciously and thereby manifest as physical pain. Feelings that have been foreclosed from awareness can lead to somatic pain, which distracts the sufferer from those feelings.

Although Dr. Sarno coined the term TMS, current literature refers to the same condition as Psychophysiologic Disorder, or PPD. For the sake of consistency, when we are discussing Dr. Sarno's contributions, the term TMS will be used; however, PPD can be used interchangeably.

In Pamela's therapy, she learned to use the pain as a "signal" that she had experienced an emotional reaction to something that had just happened. Once she had identified and experienced anger at her father, the pain disappeared. When her psychotherapy began, she was not able to tolerate experiencing "conflicting" feelings toward her father. Together, we helped her learn that she can love him and feel angry at him, simultaneously.

Defining Pain

Had Pamela not consulted with Dr. Sarno, she would probably have searched immediately for a "physical" reason for the pain that appeared suddenly and intensely at her dinner table. She might have speculated, "I probably strained my back while doing all of that hard physical work preparing for the family holiday meal." Searching for a "physical" or "structural" cause of musculoskeletal pain reflects the traditional biomedical model of disease that has dominated Western medicine for centuries, in which there is a one-to-one correspondence between physical disease or injury and pain.

That "biomedical" model has been challenged, beginning in the mid-1960s, with the research of the psychologist, Ronald Melzack, PhD. He and subsequent generations of pain researchers have substantiated that "pain" is the outcome of a perceptual process generated by the brain, even in the absence of external stimulation and/or injury and disease. Further support for this argument comes from studies of people who have "phantom limb pain," paraplegics who experience pain below the level of their severed spinal cord, and people born without limbs who feel pain in "extremities" they do not have. Numerous researchers have also demonstrated that our perception of "painful" sensations is influenced by our mood, by memories of other painful sensations, by our level of motivation, and by social and cultural learning.

We have learned from pain researchers in the past 50 years that pain is a complex subjective experience, something that Freud understood more than 100 years ago. Pain cannot be measured directly. We have to rely on the reports of the person in pain about the quality and intensity of their experience. Pain is a perceptual process that requires us to be conscious or aware. It is comprised of sensations that come from the surface of the body and the internal organs, and it can be generated in reaction to sensory images generated internally. It involves emotions because sensations pass through the limbic system in the brain where emotional memories of sensations from the past are stored. Pain perception also involves the higher brain centers (i.e., the cortex), which is associated with thinking and evaluating and complicated belief systems about sensations. Pain is a complex subjective experience that involves sensations, emotions, and thoughts.

In fact, we learn to label sensations as painful. We learn to label through our interactions with the primary care-giving others around us when we are infants, and as we continue to grow physically and develop cognitively. The care-giving others and the culture in which they live and we live give labels to sensations. The care-giving others can't see the sensation "pain"; they can only see an infant's or child's behavioral expressions in reaction to something (e.g., facial expressions, the sound of the infant's cry, the way the infant is moving around). So the mother or father, for example, interprets or evaluates behaviors of the infant to assess that he or she is in pain. They respond accordingly, depending on their assessment. So, you can begin to see how complicated this is: Because we can't measure pain objectively the way we can measure blood pressure or temperature, we have to infer that someone is in pain. Before there is language, infants and children learn the labels for their internal experiences through interactions with people who are taking care of them. Then the culture shapes how much pain is acceptable to experience. There are also gender influences that inform stereotypes about how much pain men and women can tolerate.

In the developmental process underlying our perception of pain, we also learn a set of expectations or beliefs about what constitutes another person's pain and how effectively the pain can be relieved. For example, if a young person has been in the presence of someone in acute or chronic pain or medical illness or disability, memories of those experiences become part of the developing person's memories of pain. How they experience sensations later in life will be affected by their beliefs and expectancies about how others' pain has been relieved, or not. The physician, George Engel, wrote about the significant impact of "pain memories." Melzack's research led him to conclude that a developmental process lays down the template, or the neuromatrix, for how we interpret sensations from our body, as well as sensations that are caused when we have thoughts that evoke painful or unpleasant emotions in reaction to those thoughts.

In treating pain, it is crucial to learn as much as possible about the individual's early experiences of being soothed: Did they have early experiences of being in acute pain or chronic pain? What kind of soothing was available? We now know from research on premature infants that a child who has been through a medical illness that requires multiple injections and medical treatments will be more sensitive to painful sensations later in life.

Melzack and his colleagues have produced more research that shows that there is no one center in the brain that perceives pain. In fact, pain is the result of a pattern of responses in different areas of the brain, in response to sensations that come from the outside, from the viscera, or even from our thoughts. An example of that is a session with a patient who was referred to me by Dr. Sarno because of pain in his neck. In fact, Jeff just woke up one morning with pain in his neck, and it continued for several months. He had it evaluated very carefully medically, and there was no medical or structural basis for the pain. As a result of our work in understanding his emotions at the time that the sensations of pain developed, we were able to relieve his pain. After a few months of freedom from pain, we were in a session in which we were talking about a complicated family relationship that he had had since he was a child. As he was going into the details about a recent interaction with that person, his neck started to hurt. This is a dramatic example of how thinking and talking about a situation can evoke emotions that are associated with sensations in the past, and those sensations can come up in the form of pain.

Treating Tension Myoneural Syndrome—(TMS)

First, I want to clarify that Dr. Sarno and the clinicians who work with him do not do "chronic pain management." We aim for pain relief in treating a mindbody pain condition that Dr. Sarno has delineated in his peer-reviewed publications and in his books directed at a broader audience. Dr. Sarno initiated his treatment approach 50 years ago, when he was trying to treat people for whom *all* approaches to pain relief and management had failed (e.g., surgery, hypnosis).

While Dr. Sarno did not collect data via randomized clinical trials (RCTs), the gold standard of scientific pain research, to document that his approach to pain relief works, it is illuminating to note the volume of sales of his books and the vast number of testimonials on the internet attesting to complete recovery from pain. We have many anecdotal reports of people being cured by his readings books. Activism among people who have been "cured" following his principles led to their creation, in 2009, of a website—(www.tmswiki.wetpaint.com) devoted to providing resources for people in pain and for those care for them. In addition, physicians from around the country, indeed from around the world, have been inspired by Sarno's theory and treatment approach, and have begun offering their own elaborations of it: for example, David Schechter (www.schechtermd.com), Howard Schubiner (www.unlearnyourpain.com), and Marc Sopher (www.tms-mindbodymedicine.com).

Dr. Sherman and I have the keenest respect for clinical pain research that uses randomized clinical trials (RCTs) to establish the validity of treatment interventions. We advocate research on the clinical reports made by medical, mental health, allied health care professional professionals, and people who have found relief from TMS pain. That research has already begun, in a pilot study of fibromyalgia using RCTs accepted for publication in a peer-reviewed medical journal (Schubiner & Betzold, 2012). Schubiner and his colleagues have been awarded a research grant from the National Institute of Health to expand this research.

We hope that current and succeeding generations of pain professionals and concerned lay people will promote RCTs to evaluate the methods we have found to be effective, case by case, in our clinical practices for 40 years. Pushing toward that goal, along with the aim of educating the public about TMS, in 2010, we joined a coalition of people who have been successfully treated for TMS and other health care professionals experienced in treating TMS to form a non-profit educational corporation, Psychophysiologic Disorders Association (www.ppdassociation.org).

Dr. Sarno discovered, in collaboration with the psychotherapists who were on his rehabilitation team, that his patients had difficulty acknowledging their emotions, or affects—I will use this term interchangeably with emotions going forward. It was common that these people could not feel positive or negative emotions. It was necessary to develop techniques to help people identify that they were having feelings, to name or label the feelings, and to tolerate having the feelings. Contemporary clinicians and neuroscientists refer to these processes as essential to the development of "emotional regulation" and "self-regulation."

The "technique" that I have developed over these years of treating pain is grounded in the publications of psychoanalyst researchers such as Henry Krystal (Michigan State University), his son John Krystal (Yale University), and Graeme Taylor (University of Toronto) and his colleagues in Canada. These clinician-researchers have focused on the role of emotions/affects in health and illness. In particular, their findings document the value of recognizing what we're feeling, and developing the capacity to tolerate and regulate both positive and negative emotions. Feelings/emotions/affects become problematic when we need to avoid experiencing them because they may be overwhelming. Intolerance and avoidance of emotions can be associated with physical as well as psychological illness, as documented by these and other researchers. Researchers are increasingly focusing on the significant role of emotions in health and illness, for example, in the neurobiology of fear

(Joseph LeDoux) and the neurobiology of trauma (Bessel van der Kolk and his colleagues).

My treatment approach is also influenced by 1) Allan Schore's (www.allanschore.com) integration of data from the psychoanalytic theory of development, neurobiology of attachment, and the neuroscience of emotional regulation; 2) Daniel J. Siegel's (www.drdansiegel.com) "interpersonal neurobiology," which captures the complexity of the interpenetration of the psychological and the neurobiological realms of theorizing; and 3) Wilma Bucci's (www.referentialprocess.org) research on the bodily basis of emotional and cognitive processing.

The body—disabled, disfigured, and in pain—has been the focus of my work as a clinical psychologist and psychoanalyst, beginning in 1974 with my clinical psychology internship at Rusk Institute-New York University Langone Medical Center. Learning to help children and adults cope with and surmount congenital, traumatic, and progressive loss of bodily functioning was a daunting challenge in the beginning: I had to confront my own vulnerability to the vicissitudes of life and the fear that we all have when we experience a loss of the capacity to function physically. I soon found this work compelling, and was fortunate to become a member of the psychology staff for 12 more years.

In 1998, I published "Psychic Elaboration of Musculoskeletal Pain: Ellen's Story," a detailed presentation about my work with one of Dr. Sarno's patients (in *Relational Perspectives on the Body*). The psychotherapy with Ellen compelled me to attempt to convey to an audience of psychotherapists what we discovered about pain as a mindbody disorder that could be treated effectively by the "talking cure." In this chapter, I illustrated how overwhelming emotions were related to the development of Ellen's TMS pain and discussed how we worked with these emotions in the psychotherapy process, thereby relieving her pain. While treating Dr. Sarno's patients, I developed a TMS symptom—tension headaches. As I delved into the early childhood origins of my own TMS, I refined my skills at identifying emotional sources of TMS and its equivalents. Once again, feeling compelled to reach a readership of "talking" therapists, I wrote about my personal journey, "At a Loss for Words and Feelings," in my edited book, *Bodies in Treatment: The Unspoken Dimension* (2008). I had learned that becoming aware of and tolerating feeling "hidden," "forbidden," "repressed/dissociated" emotions is the crucial entry point in recovering from TMS.

In this volume of case studies, in which we illustrate how we treat people diagnosed with TMS by Dr. Sarno, my colleague, Eric Sherman, and I hope to engage people in pain, people who are concerned about them, and professionals who treat pain. After much deliberation, we chose to focus on the stories of people in pain and, with their written contributions, illustrate how the therapist and patient collaborate to accomplish relief from TMS pain.

As psychologists, we are not qualified to make a medical diagnosis, even a psychosomatic diagnosis such as TMS. A physician makes the diagnosis through an interview and physical examination, "linking" or "re-linking" the mind and body with a diagnosis of TMS/PPD. Obviously, teamwork with the physician who makes the diagnosis is a requisite.

Let me elaborate why this teamwork is necessary. When I'm treating a patient who has been given a TMS/PPD pain diagnosis by a physician, I obtain written consent to collaborate with the physician, explaining the "rehabilitation team" approach, pioneered by Howard Rusk, MD, the father of physical rehabilitation medicine, or physiatry. I have used this philosophy effectively in collaborating with Dr. John E. Sarno since 1979.

As the treatment evolves, I learn about the person's pain pattern. If the pattern changes for the worse (e.g., the pain intensifies and/or moves to a different location), I refer them to the physician to report these changes. While I may surmise that the intensification and/or change in location are related to emotions that are being evoked and/or warded off as a result of the therapy process, the physician needs to make an assessment before we explore the hypothesized emotional "triggers" further.

When I am working with a patient who was not referred for TMS treatment, I am, nevertheless, attuned to the mindbody connection and alert to "signals" of discord that may come in the form of unpleasant/painful sensations or other medical conditions. I first recommend that the patient consult with their established physician for an evaluation. If there are "no significant findings" or the results sound ambiguous, I raise the possibility of TMS by discussing the mindbody connection and suggesting that they read material about TMS written by physicians. If they "recognize" themselves in what they read, I refer them to a physician qualified to make a TMS diagnosis.

First, I will oversimplify by saying that the treatment is implied in the diagnosis: If hidden/repressed emotions create somatic pain as a distraction or avoidance mechanism to protect the psychological self from intolerable emotional pain, then treatment must aim to identify and help the patient experience and explore those emotions. Now this appears to be very easy for many people—the ones who become pain free after reading a book on TMS. I hear stories about these people from patients and have witnessed this kind of cure among friends and family members. These people didn't need my help! How they are cured so quickly is a very interesting and important matter that I can't address further here, except to say that I've learned a good deal from treating a few of these people over the years after they've experienced a recurrence of pain that won't go away.

The people I treat have usually tried very hard to eliminate the pain and are quite discouraged and self-critical because they haven't been "successful" on their own. They often feel that they've "failed" the program, citing statistics in Dr. Sarno's books about how few people need psychotherapy. As he has described, often TMS sufferers have internalized the value "Americans" place on being independent, self-sufficient, and invulnerable and have been rewarded professionally and financially for these traits. Many of the founders of our country were people in desperate straits who had to work hard to survive. Acknowledging vulnerability and fear could have been more perilous than toughing it out. Thus, it seems to be a part of our national "character." Another large group of people with TMS have been rewarded for being nice, considerate peace-makers, for pouring oil on troubled waters, indeed for making sure that there are no troubled waters.

These admirable qualities contribute to building a robust economy and to the smooth working of our social structure. When relied on at the expense of acknowledging one's own feelings and needs, however, a consequence may be emotional and/or mindbody disorders such as TMS and its equivalents. The disavowal of dependency, vulnerability, and anger/rage contributes to overflowing emotional reservoirs of shame, fear, grief, longing, rage, and even love. In his identification of the "reservoir of rage," Dr. Sarno has demonstrated how problematic it is for many of us in our civilized western culture. Within the last few years, he has increased our awareness of the young child within who needed, and stills needs, unconditional love and acceptance. He has encouraged his patients to get to know that child through journaling and in therapy. I have brought to his attention that quite a few of my patients have discovered the frustrated, insecure adolescent who has also been unconsciously disavowed.

The treatment begins by exploring the context in which the symptom developed. Often, people do not have an awareness of the emotional impact of the physical/work/family/relationship environment in which they live because they have learned to survive and thrive by disavowing the emotions I described above. I ask for minute details, like a journalist, sometimes annoying with my "picky" questions about "who, what, when, where, and why." We learn a lot from what they can and cannot answer. My aim is to help them identify "stressors" that can lead to the overflow of an emotional reservoir into a pain symptom. For example, a 36-year-old patient recently told me that, within the past year, his father had died suddenly, he had lost his job, and separated from his life partner. While these life events would cause many of us to have overwhelming feelings, he had scant appreciation of just how stressful these events had been. Thus his therapy began.

While identifying the life events preceding the onset of the pain, I am listening intently to how the person is speaking about the event. How is my patient reacting emotionally to what they are telling me. For example, are they laughing when telling me about what sounds like an enraging/embarrassing/shaming/humiliating situation? Do they seem sad when speaking about sad matters? Can

I detect any emotion at all as they speak about a highly volatile interaction or a devastating loss? I often refer to this function of the therapist as the "emotion detector." In the initial consultation, I begin to bring the patient's attention to this dimension of their participation, carefully probing to assess the extent of their awareness and how they react to my inquiring. We often identify this as an area where they will need to do work both inside and outside of the session.

For people who have great difficulty being aware of what they are feeling about what they are saying, I work intensively on this in each session. I recommend that they take a "feeling inventory" several times during the day and evening: Ask yourself, "What am I feeling about the events that happened during the past hour? How did I feel when my supervisee didn't meet the deadline and casually brought the work into my office without acknowledging that it was late? How did I feel when our nanny called to say that she had an emergency and had to leave immediately, possibly indefinitely? How did I feel when our 16-year-old son showed up two hours past his curfew, undeniably drunk?" At the beginning of therapy, some people need to take this inventory once every hour.

As we are doing this "emotion detection" work inside and outside the sessions, we are also tracking pain levels as well as presence and absence of pain. This strategy is aimed at making links between emotions and pain symptoms. I offer a few examples to illustrate:

1) A patient had been pain-free all day but noticed that his pain started on the way to the session. I asked what he was thinking and feeling along the way. He realized that he had mixed feelings about being in the session. As we examine these feelings, his pain lessens but is not completely alleviated.

2) A patient is pain-free in the session until she starts to describe an interaction with her husband the previous night. In our discussion, we discover that she was furious with him and afraid of feeling her anger. We spend some time helping her tolerate that feeling right there in the session. As she becomes more comfortable with feeling angry, we talk about some constructive ways to use the anger to assert herself in the relationship with him. Her pain gradually subsides.

3) A patient is in excruciating pain as he enters the session and has no idea what brought on the pain the day before. We begin our search for the emotional triggers and discover that he had been dreading an upcoming phone call to his mother in which he planned to confront her in a way he had never done. As we discussed his strategy and what he was afraid would happen, his pain started to subside.

Anderson, F. S. (Ed.) (2008). *Bodies in Treatment: The Unspoken Dimension*. New York: Routledge.

Aron, L., & Anderson, F. S. (Eds.) (1998). *Relational Perspectives on the Body*. Hillsdale, NJ: The Analytic Press.

Schubiner, H., & Betzold, M. (2012). *Unlearn Your Pain*. Pleasant Ridge, MI: Mind Body Publishing.

[1] Some material in this Introduction was published earlier in digital formats. The first two paragraphs appeared in an article, "When the Mind Heals the Body," in Psych-e-News, Issue #1, January 2008 (http://198.66.163.157/docs/divisions/psychoanalysis/eNewsJan08.htm), permission granted by the Editor, Susan Parlow, PhD. Additional content was taken from an online interview in 2010, "Treating Chronic Pain" (http://www.wheretheclientis.com/2010/02/08/treating-chronic-pain-an-interview-with-frances-sommer-anderson-phd/), permission granted by the interviewer, Will Baum.

Eric Sherman

Introduction

Since 1970, John E. Sarno, MD, a physiatrist at The Rusk Institute of Rehabilitation Medicine and Professor of Rehabilitation Medicine at The New York University Langone School of Medicine, has pioneered the idea that a wide variety of pain disorders are psychophysiologic in origin. The Psychophysiologic Disorders Association (PPDA) is extending his formative contributions, now using "psychophysiologic disorders" (PPD) to encompass musculoskeletal pain and other somatic symptoms (www.ppdassociation.org .

Previously, psychophysiologic disorders were more commonly referred to as psychosomatic disorders. Such conditions develop out of the physiological reactions which accompany all emotional or psychological experiences. Psychophysiologic disorders are just one aspect of the recently energized field of mindbody medicine.

Defining TMS

Everyone is familiar with the stress-related physical symptoms that anxious students experience when preparing for exams. Among this group of young and otherwise healthy individuals, there is a disproportionate number suffering from headaches and gastrointestinal complaints prior to and during exam week. Although these students probably continue to maintain hectic schedules and appalling eating habits, once exams are over their physical complaints subside as their stress levels recede.

Another example is provided by Jerome Groopman, MD in his book, *How Doctors Think* (2007), where he describes his own experience with psychophysiologic pain. While being evaluated for hand pain, Dr. Groopman underwent a diagnostic scan that indicated possible metastatic lesions to his ribs. Dr. Groopman, himself an oncologist, recognized with horror the implications of such a finding. Metastatic lesions appear when a cancer has spread beyond its origin, auguring a bleak prognosis.

Dr. Groopman says at receiving this news he immediately felt pain and sensitivity over his ribs. Before the terrifying prospect of terminal illness, he had experienced no pain or tenderness there. Fortunately for Dr. Groopman, he soon learned that the scan has been "overread," and that he did not in fact have cancer. In a few days, he no longer felt pain and tenderness along his ribs.

These examples demonstrate the cornerstone of Dr. Sarno's theoretical and clinical approach to treating psychophysiologic pain disorders: Emotional distress can be directly translated into physical pain, even without permanent alterations in the structure or functioning of the affected part of the body.

Dr. Sarno published numerous papers and a series of books on psychophysiologic pain disorders. His most recent is *The Divided Mind* (2006). In his writing, Dr. Sarno identifies Tension Myoneural Syndrome (TMS) as a benign, psychophysiologic process in which mild ischemia of postural muscles, nerves, and a variety of tendons is initiated by dynamic psychological factors.

What does that mean? Myoneural refers both to the functional and structural relationships between muscles (myo-) and nerves (neural). Nerves transmit electrical signals to muscles, commanding them to contract or relax. Ischemia describes a condition of reduced blood flow or circulation to a particular area. Dynamic psychological factors are psychological forces that operate outside of an individual's awareness yet still affect that individual's behavior, just like an odorless and colorless gas causing baffling physical reactions. Therefore, TMS is a psychophysiologic pain disorder in which emotional experiences, which may be partially or completely out of a person's awareness, produce ischemia or reduced blood flow to the postural muscles, resulting in mild oxygen deprivation and pain.

The overlapping relationships between blood flow, emotional experiences, and physiological reactions are immediately recognizable in the everyday phenomena of erections and blushing. Embarrassment is accompanied by increased circulation to the face and neck, and when a person is frightened, the blood drains from his face and he acquires a ghostly pallor. Sexual arousal redirects blood flow to the penis, which is actually a muscle, and an erection ensues. If that same person experiences fear or self-consciousness, blood flow to the penis is reduced and the man cannot sustain his erection. The interaction among emotional experiences, blood flow, and myoneural activity is the same psychophysiologic process involved in TMS.

Dr. Sarno described TMS as a physical disorder characterized by pain and/or other neural signs and symptoms affecting a variety of musculoskeletal locations. We use the term *pathophysiology* to refer to how a disease or malfunction arises from abnormalities in the structure or functioning of bodily systems. The pathophysiology of TMS involves the circulatory system.

While some researchers and clinicians in the field of mindbody medicine have recently challenged Dr. Sarno's idea that the pathophysiology of TMS involves the circulatory system (Schubiner, 2010), our clinical material is based on the psychoeducational treatment model first developed by Dr. Sarno. Further research will eventually elucidate the physiological basis of TMS pain symptomatology. Although the scientific questions surrounding the pathophysiology of TMS are still unresolved, this psychologically-based treatment approach has been demonstrated to be highly effective.

Dr. Sarno emphasized that the pain is real; it is not imaginary or "in the patient's head," as is sometimes misconstrued by physicians and analytically oriented clinicians. For example, few would misunderstand diarrhea as "fake," imaginary, or "just in the patient's head," simply because it resulted from a "nervous stomach."

Even though TMS is a mindbody disorder, the subjective experience of the pain is indistinguishable from pain originating from organic conditions such as injuries, tumors, and infections, even though the pathophysiology responsible for the syndrome is psychologically induced.

Dr. Sarno conceptualized the pain symptomatology as a self-protective reaction or a defense against recognizing and experiencing intolerable affects, not the result of structural damage or disease. So, when a herniated disc is diagnosed as the cause of someone's pain and disability, a psychophysiologic disorder is misdiagnosed and physical treatments not only fail, but also serve to intensify the symptomatology.

Appropriate treatment is delayed or denied, and iatrogenic, or physician-induced, debility develops. The person becomes increasingly preoccupied with the pain symptomatology. Now every bodily sensation echoes and confirms the doctor's dire assessment, reinforcing his own sense of being permanently damaged.

Dr. Sarno reported that analytically-oriented psychotherapy is essential for cure in the 20-25% of cases which do not respond sufficiently to his psychoeducational program, the first step in treating TMS patients.

Of great interest is that large numbers of people have experienced complete and sustained resolution of their pain symptomatology after reading one of Dr. Sarno's books. They resume all of their previous activities without developing new or worsening pain symptomatology. These results are important in theorizing on the nature of the psychophysiologic process and what is required to reverse it. Clearly, the acquisition of information about the process must be therapeutic. Again, it worked for Dr. Groopman as well; his rib pain vanished once he received the good news that he did not have cancer.

(Mis)Diagnosing TMS

All too often, physicians who treat pain, psychotherapists, and even people struggling with musculoskeletal pain attribute physical problems exclusively to anatomical defects, thereby "medicalizing" them. In our failure to recognize the crucial role psychodynamic factors play in the development of persistent musculoskeletal pain, we undermine the effectiveness of clinicians and inadvertently deprive people of beneficial treatment.

According to the website of The American Academy of Pain Medicine (12/12), pain disorders are a major public health problem in the Western world. "The total annual incremental cost of health care due to pain ranges from $560 billion to $635 billion (in 2010 dollars) in the United States, which combines the medical costs of pain care and the economic costs related to disability days and lost wages and productivity." (http://www.painmed.org/patientcenter/facts_on_pain.aspx#refer .

Many physicians in all specialties have been trained that structural abnormalities identified on x-ray or imaging studies are the cause of pain, despite the lack of correlation of the patient's signs or symptoms with the study findings. Experience with thousands of people with these pain manifestations has demonstrated, by successful treatment, that they are not caused by the structural abnormalities (e.g., herniated disc), but by TMS. In fact, individuals with these same structural abnormalities can in some cases be entirely asymptomatic and unaware of any problem, while others are significantly debilitated.

What follows is a common experience among people seeking medical evaluation for their musculoskeletal pain symptomatology. This particular individual suffered from chronic, excruciating neck pain. After reviewing the MRIs of the patient's neck and spine, the orthopedist informed him, "Your neck looks fine, but your back is a train wreck." The patient, an avid sportsman, had never experienced any back pain.

Herniated discs are routinely detected on asymptomatic patients undergoing CT scanning for unrelated conditions. However, in symptomatic patients, the very same findings will be the basis for establishing a pain diagnosis. People's responses to identical treatments for the same condition vary widely, often in ways that bear no causal relationship to the pathophysiology implicated by the physical diagnosis. Both medical specialists and mental health professionals often only respond to somatic symptoms as medical conditions, which are consequently misunderstood and mismanaged by both disciplines.

Jerome Groopman, MD (2002) debunked the rationale for many common surgical procedures to treat back pain. He observes that pain relief is often so unsatisfactory that other procedures with a similarly abysmal track record would be outlawed, and certainly not underwritten by insurance companies.

Richard Deyo, MD(2004), an internist who has extensively reviewed medical and surgical approaches to back pain, concludes also that Dr. Sarno's diagnostic and therapeutic practices can be effective and are insufficiently utilized by medical practitioners.

TMS: An Historical Perspective

Although Dr. Sarno is unique among medical specialists in his appreciation of the psychophysiologic nature of chronic pain, his work in this area has long been foreshadowed by many psychoanalytic thinkers. Freud first observed in 1895 in *Studies on Hysteria* (2005) that "intractable physical symptoms can be divorced from their biological origins." The contemporary psychoanalytic theorist Joyce McDougall points out that physical and affective pain can be "confused or substituted for one another as part of psychic defense." She has advanced the related position that "all emotion is psychosomatic" (Aron & Anderson, 1998).

Similar ideas about the intrinsic relationship between emotions and physiology were delineated by Walter Cannon in his naturalistic experiments on gastric acid production and emotional stimulation, almost a century earlier.

Masters and Johnson (1966) showed what everyone, especially the pornography industry, has known forever: Sexual fantasies alone can directly and immediately lead to the physiological changes evident in erection and vaginal lubrication. Essentially, sexual arousal is a normal application of the very same psychophysiologic mechanisms underlying TMS.

Despite our access to seminal contributions on psychophysiologic conditions, musculoskeletal pain and other mindbody disorders continue to be relatively ignored as a psychophysiologic disorder by both the medical and mental health communities. As a result of this collective neglect, we lack the breadth of experience with this topic to discuss it in a nuanced manner.

With respect to etiology, psychophysiologic pain disorders are not homogeneous entities; one size does not fit all. Some people suffering from TMS drastically resolve internal conflicts over aggressive and dependent wishes by developing musculoskeletal pain as a compelling distraction from these disruptive feelings. For others, pain symptomatology develops when a person cannot put his feelings into words and is forced to rely on a body language of physical sensations to express these experiences.

Another group of people with psychophysiologic pain disorders dissociates, or severs the experience of emotional pain from the conscious awareness of it. Their bodies become the burial grounds for these disconnected feelings. Their pain symptomatology simultaneously contains and conceals these dissociated emotions.

Secondary gain refers to concrete benefits or "rewards" for suffering, such as obtaining extra attention or being exempt from responsibilities. Rarely do the lures of secondary gain appeal to the patients we treat. Complicating this discussion even further is the fact that the bulk of research on pain has been conducted on cancer patients, post-surgical patients, and individuals receiving benefits from Worker's Compensation. In contrast to this last subgroup of people, the overwhelming majority of Dr. Sarno's patients continue to work, often despite debilitating pain and/or sedation from narcotic analgesics prescribed for pain relief.

The (Mis)Treatment of Pain Symptomatology

Whether musculoskeletal pain is conceptualized as a psychophysiologic condition or not determines its fate as a symptom, a complaint, or a communication in the treatment situation.

For many psychotherapists, regardless of their theoretical leanings, pain symptomatology is fundamentally unrelated to a person's character structure, interpersonal relationships, level of maturity, or psychodynamics. On the contrary, musculoskeletal pain is more often regarded as an unfortunate complication in their lives: the inevitable consequences of aging, injury, or illness.

Both medical and mental health clinicians would agree, of course, that emotional distress must accompany any experience of physical pain and its associated losses and limitations in activity. In fact, when people deny such reactions, we generally become suspicious. It is widely recognized that anxiety and depression will exacerbate an individual's experience of pain. Nevertheless, for many psychotherapists and physicians, pain symptomatology still remains essentially a medical event, which can be favorably or unfavorably influenced by psychological factors. But for these health care providers, it is neither caused nor resolved by elucidating these very same emotional factors.

Because of my work with Dr. Sarno, my treatment of people suffering from musculoskeletal pain, in contrast to mainstream thinking about the diagnosis and treatment of musculoskeletal pain, is guided by the idea that pain symptomatology develops in response to intolerable emotional experiences, not the other way around.

Pain functions as a compelling distraction, deflecting an individual's attention away from unbearably frightening or disruptive internal experiences. Pain is also an expression of body language, which is the forerunner of words and the mother tongue of our internal experiences.

So, our task as clinicians treating people with psychophysiologic disorders is to understand how and why the body has become their preferred mode of communication. We ask ourselves, why has this person never learned to speak in sentences? Why is the patient reverting to the mother tongue of body language?

When individuals can neither identify nor verbalize their emotional experiences, they often develop psychophysiologic conditions, including musculoskeletal pain. These seminal observations about the relationship between the development of psychophysiologic disorders and the inability to identify, differentiate, and verbalize affects were formulated by Peter Sifneos (1973) in his description of alexithymia. Essentially, patients experience and express their emotions through a body language of physical sensations instead of symbolically representing them in words.

Obviously, such profound differences in our ways of thinking about pain symptomatology influence the development and application of techniques for treating people with psychophysiologic disorders, including musculoskeletal pain. What are the changes in technique that come from this different way of thinking, and what is their rationale?

Technical Considerations

Although a physician must establish the diagnosis of TMS, physicians, mental health professionals, and people suffering with musculoskeletal pain all need to be attuned to this possibility when someone develops musculoskeletal pain and other mindbody conditions.

Many people suffering with psychophysiologic pain have undergone prior treatment, often with analytically-oriented clinicians. Those who began treatment with musculoskeletal pain introduced their problem with references to old injuries or the onslaught of aging, all corroborated by numerous specialists and imaging studies.

Other people first developed musculoskeletal pain during the course of treatment, although a careful review of their histories will often reveal prolonged bouts with other conditions more commonly accepted as psychophysiologic in origin (e.g., headaches, hives, spastic colon, and so on). The onset of musculoskeletal pain is explained in terms of a recent injury or the aggravation of an old injury. The specialists' opinions and the results of the imaging studies are cited to document the source of their pain and legitimize its effects upon their lives.

Infrequently, the question is raised (more often by the person suffering from musculoskeletal pain): Could this pain be symptomatic of a psychophysiologic condition? The individual will observe that the pain fluctuates in severity, almost disappearing while on vacation, for example, but escalating just before an important business meeting. Or, the person notices that the pain precludes sexual activity but never interferes with other prolonged and strenuous activities.

Typically, the therapist responds to these reports with comments such as: "You prefer to believe your condition is caused by emotional stress so you don't have to think about the fact that you're aging and you're not a kid anymore," or "Your pain may come and go and you're focusing on that to avoid taking in what the doctors told you about your herniated disc and how you now have to modify your lifestyle."

Clearly, these interventions make sense if pain is conceptualized as an exclusively medical phenomenon, lying beyond the legitimate realm of psychotherapy. Thus, the persistence of pain is acknowledged sadly as yet another example of life's essential unfairness.

Psychotherapists frequently try to explore the emotionally-tinged ideas a person might privately hold about his pain symptomatology. Some people may believe that they are suffering in order to atone for their angry and destructive wishes, or they hope their obvious infirmity will placate powerful enemies and insure their continued dependency. Although this therapeutic approach inadvertently acknowledges a relationship between emotional experience and pain symptomatology, the individual's emotional experiences are still seen as reactive instead of causal with respect to the development of musculoskeletal pain.

At this point, a therapist who is unfamiliar with mindbody disorders might suggest that such personal theories about the pain bolster that individual's sense of invincibility. The idea that pain arises directly from emotional conflicts effectively trumps the even more feared notion that the body itself is irreparably damaged. However, this line of reasoning is often disparaged as a self-consoling fantasy aimed at denying overwhelming feelings of loss and helplessness.

Much useful work can result when the treatment continues along these lines. However, the primacy of intolerable affective states in the development of pain is still unappreciated in the above model. Pain is still understood to be an experience that happens from without, as opposed to arising from within the patient.

When people are referred to me for treatment, I tell them that I will not work with them if they are currently involved in individual psychotherapy with another therapist. Not infrequently, the current therapist will express genuine perplexity and ask, "Can't you just treat the back problem, and I'll continue to work with him on those other issues?" Although some of these therapists might fear losing income, it seems that the majority of them don't appreciate the fact that "the hip bone's connected to the thigh bone." They don't fully realize that emotional difficulties underlying the development of musculoskeletal pain cannot be simply subtracted away from the rest of someone's personality.

The medicalization of musculoskeletal pain further compromises the psychotherapist's ability to treat the person suffering with TMS or other mindbody disorders. If the mental health professional regards the person's pain symptomatology as the result of a herniated disc, for example, then the thrust of the work must be directed towards understanding the various ways that someone mourns his loss or struggles against accepting it.

If someone exercises, then the behavior is branded as self-defeating and non-compliant, a defiant expression of his refusal to mourn and accept the losses that accompany his medical condition. Or, the patient is viewed as masochistic and passive when he doesn't exhaustively pursue every medical option, including contradictory and illogical ones.

When someone grieves and accepts the permanence of his physical losses, the treatment is proceeding smoothly. However, if the individual complains incessantly about his pain, then he is trying to make the therapist feel useless. Of course the therapist is useless; he can't fix structurally damaged bodies. In this model, the therapist can only help someone come to terms with his losses, but the individual's demands relocate their relationship into an arena which is not within the scope of his practice.

Resistance is a term which describes the approach-avoidance behavior that we all exhibit whenever we're seeking help with a problem. Whether it's canceling the dental appointment, or vowing to begin that diet tomorrow, even the most single-minded individual displays some apprehension during his quest for self-improvement. It is only our belief that our plan of action will ultimately benefit us that enables us to tolerate the anxiety we inevitably develop whenever we initiate positive changes. When I encounter resistance to accepting the TMS diagnosis, I refocus the person's attention on the relationship between his intolerance of emotional experience and the onset of physical suffering. I question not only why the he tries to make me feel useless, but also why he is not utilizing my expertise to help him identify and understand the very emotional experiences which bring on the pain in the first place.

Intense preoccupations with pain symptomatology and insistence upon finding a physical explanation for their condition distance people from their underlying emotional experience in the very same way pain distracts them from unbearable feelings. Instead, I reframe anguished concern about one's health as a cry for help, a poignant appeal for a loved one's rapt attention and caring.

Oddly, psychotherapists often feel comfortable treating headaches and abdominal pain as psychophysiologic disorders. Many people have often described psychophysiologic musculoskeletal pain as "a headache in my back" or "it's like I'm having a stomach ache in my back."

Why both the mental health and medical communities have resisted recognizing musculoskeletal pain as a psychophysiologic disorder is a subject for another book.

The therapist who medicalizes pain can accept someone's expressions of anger, sadness, and fear as appropriate responses to his condition. Unfortunately, this same therapist fails to appreciate how that person's experience of these feelings of anger, sadness, and fear directly contributes to the pain symptomatology in the first place.

Once a therapist recognizes musculoskeletal pain as a mindbody disorder, then the goals of treatment change. Complaints of pain are no longer disregarded as static in the background, but are appreciated instead as distress signals originating from the person's inner life. The emphasis in therapy shifts from mourning the physical losses associated with pain symptomatology to developing a richer and more extensive emotional vocabulary for coping with painful emotional states. This process resembles frustrated parents exhorting their toddlers to "use your words" instead of throwing a tantrum. Children whose language skills have not developed sufficiently to express their emotional distress in words revert to the primitive body language of a tantrum to communicate their needs. In some ways, TMS is an adult version of the toddler's fit, an agonizing mismatch between an individual's distress and his ability to convey it to others in words. A patient once characterized treatment for TMS as "translating body language into the heartache or emotional pain that created it in the first place."

We instruct people to utilize the pain symptomatology as a signal to guide their introspection. Instead of asking himself, "Did I just move the wrong way?" "Did I lift something too heavy?" or "Did something just snap or pull?" the person is encouraged to observe, "What was I just feeling emotionally, right before the pain started?"

Once people are involved in treatment, they spontaneously observe, as a typical example, that the pain began while they were sitting and reading, and therefore no physical activity could possibly explain the onset of the pain at that particular time. Similarly, when an individual can identify an affect or differentiate it from other ones, we inquire in detail about the accompanying physical sensations. The inextricable connection between emotional experiences and physical sensations is constantly highlighted, and the individual becomes adept at utilizing his knowledge about this relationship as a tool to resolve his own pain symptomatology.

Some people have reported that during previous courses of treatment, their irritable bowel syndrome, for example, significantly improved or completely resolved. Unfortunately, even though the individual extensively examined his affective experience, a causal relationship was not demonstrated between his feelings and the development of the symptoms. Therefore, the person cannot utilize such knowledge as a resource for dealing with these symptoms in the future and comes to regard the improvement as a non-specific benefit of treatment.

People suffering with psychophysiologic pain disorders will frequently remark, "I couldn't stomach it," "It's all on my shoulders," "My mother-in-law got my back up," or "I wouldn't put my foot down." They are often quite surprised by their reliance on somatic imagery to describe their feelings. They are even more surprised by the difficulty they experience when trying to put these feelings into words. When asked "How does that make you feel?" they will often respond with intellectualizations, report increased pain or other uncomfortable physical sensations, draw a blank, or demure with a "You know what I mean."

My work with people diagnosed with TMS regularly confirms Sifneos' findings on alexithymia: When an individual can't put his feelings into words, he defaults to body language to express these sentiments.

Disconnecting and Reconnecting with Feelings

People with TMS often describe events in their lives with either no apparent emotional reaction or convey an emotional reaction that doesn't fit with the experience they are describing. For example, they may describe brutal treatment from important figures in their lives while grinning broadly. A common example of this tendency is the individual who relates tragic events with unflappability.

When a person's attention is directed to this behavior, his surprise is immediately followed with rationalizations as to why he shouldn't experience or express such feelings: "You can't expect me to cry about it all the time," or "You can't go ranting and raving in civilized society!"

Many people fear that if they dare experience a feeling,

they will inevitably act on it. If you recognize a feeling, it becomes real. Therefore, experiencing, recognizing, or expressing certain emotions pose a threat, which can be obliterated from their awareness by physical pain.

Contrary to the widely held notion that emotional inhibition is ubiquitous among people with TMS, there is a sub-group of these individuals who openly (and sometimes inappropriately) express anger to important and powerful figures in their lives.

Although some people will consciously stifle their rage, they simultaneously express confidence that the target of their anger could readily accept their feelings. Perhaps this discrepancy between expectations and behavior belies a doubt the patient disavows.

However, what is more distressing for these individuals is the private, internal, emotional experience of feelings. They are often more troubled by the recognition of their own angry feelings than the ensuing disruptions caused by their actions. For many of these people, emotional experience, regardless of its nature, is fraught with dangers from which they seek refuge through physical pain. When emotional experience undermines both the person's sense of self-continuity and self-cohesion, it becomes intolerable. Ambivalent feelings can call into question both the authenticity and durability of the person's emotional experience. If someone cannot maintain a sense of integrity while experiencing such unruly feelings, then these experiences must be dissociated from awareness. They must be banished to a place where they can no longer be recognized and experienced as emotions, to the realm of bodily sensations.

In these instances, musculoskeletal pain and other psychophysiologic disorders operate like brown-outs, which avert blackouts. The patient sheds overwhelming and disruptive emotional experiences by sequestering them in the body. Thus, the patient's self-continuity is preserved through this dimming of awareness.

Bessel van der Kolk (1994), a pre-eminent trauma researcher and theorist, put it epigrammatically: "The body keeps the score." Significantly, many people report that the emotional distress they experience as their pain symptomatology improves is more unbearable than the physical pain, which initially brought them into treatment.

The inability to tolerate feelings can resemble hurling a hot potato, instead of holding it in your hand. If you fear that the first licks of heat threaten to burn a hole in your hand, it is imperative that you get rid of the potato in order to protect yourself from injury. If, on the other hand, you don't fear devastating injury from the heat, but instead can tolerate the temporary pain, then you don't have to respond impulsively. You can set it down to cool and eat it later, instead of having to toss it into the trash. If you fear your feelings will overwhelm you, you have no choice but to discharge them on an emergency basis, often by developing psychophysiologic symptoms.

There are myriad reasons why feelings might be experienced as unbearable. Feelings that challenge your sense of self-worth and acceptability may provoke drastic, protective measures. One person may believe that, to be a loyal spouse, he should never be attracted to anyone but his mate. When he inevitably experiences these forbidden feelings, he must treat them like an emotional hot potato to avoid damaging his self-esteem.

Another may fear that a sufficiently sturdy firewall does not exist between feelings and actions, so any feeling becomes Mrs. O'Leary's cow, whose random hoof shrug ignited the great Chicago fire.

And yet a third person may not be able to put his feelings into words, so they remain meaningless and cannot be understood and mastered. Such experiences then loom as mysterious and unpredictable forces that can disrupt someone's integrity, almost like demonic possession.

Several steps can be taken to help people learn to identify what they are feeling and learn to tolerate the feeling, and therefore not develop physical symptoms. To the extent the person does not regard his feelings as the inevitable and automatic precursors to action, then such feelings become more bearable because they are now under his control. Having this control allows the person to reflect on his feelings and have the option for more nuanced responses. If he can explain his feelings in words, then they no longer possess the power to overwhelm, like an earthquake, which erupts from within. When the rumblings are identified as an earthquake, he can seek shelter. If the tremors are not recognized as such—that is, he cannot describe the sensations in words and meaning cannot be ascribed to them—he doesn't know what to do. He either thrashes about madly or becomes paralyzed by fear and indecision. Neither response will help him cope with the impending danger. The enemy that is seen is less dangerous than the enemy that is unseen. In the case of psychophysiologic pain, when feelings can be identified, put into words, and given meaning, they are less likely to be relegated to or remain in a dissociated state, which can often be a precondition for the development of psychophysiologic pain symptomatology. And when patients can accept that their feelings are just private, internal emotional experiences and not indicators of morality, sanity, or virtue, then they can tolerate the anti-social and politically incorrect impulses that seize all of us—without risking a loss of self-esteem or a withdrawal of love from important others. When affect tolerance is increased, the patient has more adaptive options available to him for dealing with these feelings, instead of developing psychophysiologic pain or other symptoms.

My clinical experience with people with musculoskeletal pain and other psychophysiologic disorders is seldom unique. During previous courses of treatment, many of these people have learned about their tendencies towards intellectualizing, people-pleasing, and perfectionism. They have also observed how they avoid experiencing their feelings by dissociating and becoming intensely preoccupied with their physical symptoms. Some of them have come to recognize the difficulties they experience in identifying feelings and putting them into words. What distinguishes the approach we use with these individuals is the continuous emphasis on the critical role the dissociation of affective experience plays in the development of pain symptomatology. We systematically highlight the many ways these people tend to exclude their own emotional experiences from awareness, leaving their bodies to fill the void.

The role of emotional disconnection in the etiology of psychophysiologic pain disorders and other mindbody dysfunctions can best be understood through example. Anniversary reactions reveal the inner workings of dissociation.

A woman reported to me with considerable panic that she was bleeding in between her periods. She claimed that her periods were so regular, "the atomic clock could be set" according to her menstrual cycle. Her periods were so regular that she knew she was pregnant if she was "only twenty seconds late." The patient was convinced that her bleeding was symptomatic of some dreaded disease. She feared that a cancer had eaten its way through her uterine wall, causing the irregular bleeding. She attempted to schedule an emergency appointment with her gynecologist. He was away on vacation, and she was referred to a colleague. Since she had never consulted with this gynecologist before, he asked her all the usual questions pertinent to a first visit. When he asked her if she had ever been pregnant, she replied, "I had a miscarriage last year." As she was answering the question, she remembered that the miscarriage had occurred exactly one year ago, to the day. She commented to herself, "My uterus must be shedding tears of blood for the baby I didn't cry over."

After the gynecologist completed his examination, he informed her that he couldn't find anything that could explain her abnormal bleeding. He suggested they regard this episode of irregular bleeding as a hormonal blip, and if her next period occurred on schedule, to forget about it. If the bleeding persisted, then he would recommend they initiate a million-dollar workup. Her next period came as expected.

Unlike denial or repression, the patient maintained cognitive awareness that she miscarried on a particular day. What she failed to remember, but her "body kept the score," was the grief she experienced around the pregnancy loss.

In another example of an anniversary reaction, an individual who enjoyed long-standing relief from TMS suddenly developed incapacitating back pain, unrelated to any unusual physical activity. Later that day, she received a call from her sister, who wanted to commiserate over their mother's death, a year ago that very day. Again, this individual was completely aware of her mother's death. However, she was disconnected from her own overpowering feelings of loss, which she would have experienced with intolerable intensity, if her memory and experience were an integrated whole. Physical pain was substituted for emotional pain until the patient found the words to express her feelings of loss. The pain gradually subsided over several days as the patient recognized how bereft and angry she felt as a result of her mother's death.

Truly, as one individual remarked, the role of psychotherapy in the treatment of musculoskeletal pain is to find the words to translate body language into the heartache that first created it.

Clinical Implications: Two Case Histories

The following two case histories highlight the clinical implications for diagnosis and treatment when the mind and the body are viewed as two separate and distinct (or unrelated/disconnected) entities.

Liam[2] was almost 34 years old when he initially presented for treatment of severe, psychophysiologic back pain. Liam is a classic primogenitor—the oldest of four boys. He is the much-adored "Christ-grandchild" in a large, extended European family. Liam describes himself as an army brat. He is dazzlingly fluent in three languages; he oozes the easy charm and self-assurance of someone who has literally seen the world. Liam sees himself as one whose case leaps out from the pages of Dr. Sarno's books. A high achiever and well-liked by everyone, Liam never has an unkind word for anyone—not at least out loud.

Liam's first episode of disabling back pain occurred on a flight home from a vacation. Unexpectedly, he ran into his former fiancée's best girlfriend on the flight. The woman updated Liam with news that his former fiancée was engaged to another man and would be marrying later that year. Although nothing was explicitly stated, Liam "just knew" this woman noticed he was unattached, and "couldn't wait" to tell his former fiancée the good news about the pathetic state of his love life. When Liam helped the woman stow her baggage in an overhead bin, he was stricken with severe back spasms, causing him to fall to the floor in the aisle of the plane. At the time, Liam concluded that he must have "pulled something." Braced by several stiff drinks, he endured the 3½ hour flight back, hoping that his back pain was just a freak occurrence. After all, he was an extremely healthy, very athletic 30-year-old. How could anything as innocuous as stowing a small suitcase result in such pain?

After several agonizing days at home, Liam consulted a physician who referred him to an orthopedist. The orthopedist ordered an MRI, which revealed a herniation at the third and fourth lumbar vertebrae. The orthopedist subsequently prescribed conservative treatment with bed rest, anti-inflammatory drugs and possible physical therapy (depending on Liam's response to the other recommendations).

Liam's condition in fact barely improved, and he was referred to a physical therapist for more aggressive treatment. He gradually improved and discontinued the physical therapy on his own. He remained entirely asymptomatic for almost four years before suffering a recurrence of back pain.

Considering his previous history, the orthopedists he consulted this time all recommended surgery. When he learned, however, that his latest MRI was indistinguishable from the original, he questioned the need for surgery. He surmised: If after all nothing is changed on the X-ray, and I remained asymptomatic for four years without surgery, why isn't it reasonable to assume the same thing could happen again? He also wondered if there might not be another cause for his pain, since there was no interval change noted on the MRI. After all, he had been both symptomatic and asymptomatic, yet the x-ray findings remained the same, regardless of his physical condition. To a man, the doctors dismissed his question and invoked his previous history of back pain as the basis for recommending surgery.

Liam systematically availed himself of almost every known alternative treatment, with varying degrees of improvement. While searching a bookstore for yet more information, he happened upon several of Dr. Sarno's books. Reading them, he recognized himself on almost every page. He realized in hindsight that his first episode of back pain was almost certainly precipitated by an avalanche of unresolved feelings surrounding his broken engagement.

Liam consulted Dr. Sarno, who referred him to a psychologist experienced in treating patients with TMS. It took the better part of a year before Liam enjoyed any improvement in his pain symptomatology. He was at that point able to come to an understanding of why it had been necessary for certain emotional conflicts to be banned from his conscious awareness.

Although Liam was consciously aware of intensely angry feelings towards his father, he was deeply ashamed of having these feelings. Adding to his shame was his belief that he was the only one in his family who experienced such feelings of hatred. On the rare occasions when Liam voiced protest or disagreement with his father, the father would dramatically express his outrage and emotional injury. The father's behavior coerced the son into recanting his blasphemous sentiments. Of course, he erroneously interpreted his mother's passivity and his brothers' silence as support for the father.

Like many people suffering from psychophysiologic pain syndromes, Liam frequently plays the role of the hero who saves the day. He is the member of the family that everyone else looks up to. He is the consummate caretaker. He has been in training for this role since his earliest childhood. Growing up, he translated for his parents and explained American culture to them. He interceded for his brothers when cultural clashes inevitably occurred. And he consoled his mother in her marital disappointments by being the best son any mother could ever ask for. Liam's self-esteem was entirely predicated upon successfully taking care of others, especially at his own expense.

Most people, as well as those struggling with TMS, are in conflict over their very human wishes to be loved and cherished. For many of them, dependency is an expression of lovability. For others, dependency represents a shameful and terrifying loss of control. So the very same experience of yearning to be taken care of can result in feelings of being cherished and special, or burdensome and unlovable. Therefore, it is essential to examine these multifaceted feelings during treatment for musculoskeletal pain and other psychophysiologic disorders.

That Liam disavowed his own needs did not mean they didn't exist. They simply operated out of his awareness and influenced his behavior like an odorless, colorless gas. In taking care of others, Liam was able to reassure himself and others, proclaiming: "I have no needs. I am not the dependent one. I can take care of everyone else." He identified with the recipients of his caretaking and thereby vicariously gratified his own dependency needs. His physical suffering also enabled him to circumvent his prohibitions against directly recognizing and experiencing his own wishes for caretaking. He could now convince himself that he needed help because he was sick, not because he longed to be taken care of and released from certain responsibilities.

Before treatment, the acknowledgement of these wishes would have been anathema to Liam. The mere existence of these wishes, even on a private, internal, emotional basis could only mean that he was weak and despicable, unworthy of anyone's love. So he contorted both his sense of self and his body to prevent the recognition of his dependency needs. His survival demanded that these feelings be obliterated or camouflaged. His psychophysiologic pain certainly accomplished this.

As treatment progressed, it became clearer that if Liam were to believe that other members of his family shared his feelings towards his father, then he could see that his anger represented a legitimate reaction to his father's tyranny, not a sign of a son's disloyalty and ingratitude. When Liam finally mustered the courage to question his brothers and his mother about their reactions to his father, all of them freely expressed fantasies of homicidal rage towards him. His saintly mother confided how she secretly wished to strike his father across the side of his head with a hot iron, and one of his altar boy brothers shared how he often thought about pushing his father in front of a bus.

Once he was able to recognize the father's abuse, however, Liam began to feel self-loathing for having failed to protect his mother and brothers. For a long time, it had become more comfortable for Liam to feel shame for his angry feelings than shame for his scared and helpless feelings. Eventually, Liam developed compassion for himself. He was able to maintain his self-esteem by recognizing that it was not weakness, but the natural dependence of a child that made him vulnerable to the feelings of inadequacy.

Liam has remained completely asymptomatic for more than three years, despite having experienced a series of tragic events during that time. According to Liam, "I can now feel shitty, without feeling like I'm shit." And because Liam can merely feel "shitty,", he doesn't experience back pain.

* * *

In another instance, Abner[3], a 35-year-old man, presented with a several-month history of severe low back and right sciatic pain. He had already seen several orthopedists who recommended disc surgery for herniations of the third and fourth lumbar vertebrae, as shown on an MRI.

He was frightened just by the prospect of surgery. If that weren't enough, he was also well aware of the disappointing results of friends and relatives who had undergone similar procedures. Abner clearly appeared anguished, and his physical activity was significantly limited.

One member of Abner's church was alarmed by the contrast between Abner's current physical state and his former hard-driving, indefatigable style. This acquaintance spoke to Abner and learned the specifics of his back pain and the recommendations for surgery. He told Abner about his own struggle with incapacitating back pain. He explained how his symptoms began to improve after consulting with John Sarno, MD. He described how Dr. Sarno considered back pain a psychophysiologic symptom, not the aftermath of a structural defect in the spine. At this point, Abner was desperate and willing to consider anything.

Abner pursued his friend's recommendation to see Dr. Sarno. Being an extremely intelligent person and able to master complex and novel information, Abner quickly grasped Dr. Sarno's central premise that disavowed anger plays a critical role in the development of back pain. The unique problem for Abner was that he didn't consider himself emotionally inhibited.

In fact, Abner and those closest to him would agree that Abner was angry most of the time. They knew him to be a hot-headed, argumentative man, who not only sought out and provoked confrontations, but also seemed to relish them regardless of the outcome.

Therefore, Abner feared Dr. Sarno's approach would not apply to his case. He began to resign himself to surgery. However, the very fear of surgery helped him overcome his misgivings about the accuracy of Dr. Sarno's diagnosis. He accepted that his pain symptomatology was a psychophysiologic disorder, and reluctantly followed Dr. Sarno's recommendation for individual psychotherapy.

Abner, a highly engaging and dauntingly articulate man, began treatment boasting in meticulous detail about his most recent angry outbursts. He was genuinely baffled how someone like him could possibly be denying angry feelings, and so questioned how he could ever be helped by treatment. As the therapy proceeded, it became apparent that Abner reacted anaphylactically to common indignities we all endure in the course of a day.

Though still unconvinced that treatment could help him, Abner was nevertheless able to develop insight into his disproportionately intense reactions to what even he agreed were generally trivial provocations. He became curious about why he felt impelled to "kill houseflies with howitzers," even when the potential benefits could hardly justify the amount of time, effort, and energy he invested in these battles.

Abner began to observe that whenever he perceived slights, he experienced the other person as "dissing" him, essentially conveying to Abner that he was unimportant and unworthy of consideration. On his own, Abner realized quickly that these feelings were painfully familiar to him. During his childhood his own mother had been so preoccupied with her mother's ill health and needs for caretaking that she often neglected Abner's emotional needs, frequently delegating his care to others. When Abner, craving his mother's attention, would naturally protest, he was scolded for being selfish, thinking about himself instead of his sick grandmother.

To make matters worse, Abner's father, a businessman, was extremely grandiose. The father would buttress his precarious sense of self by subjecting the family to gassy accounts of his derring-do in the business world. Whenever Abner would seek his father's attention on these occasions, he would be reprimanded for not listening. If Abner failed to support his parents' narcissism, he would be punished for being selfish and self-centered. The cruel irony of this warped family dynamic infuriated Abner. He railed against the injustice of a child having to sacrifice himself in order to protect his parents. His understanding of this dilemma deepened as Abner realized that this self-sacrifice was essential for his own survival. If he didn't follow the rules, he would be less likely to receive even the crumbs of parental attention he barely subsisted on.

With this realization, Abner revised his sense of himself in a significant manner. Although he was often explosive towards others, he now appreciated how extremely inhibited he was when it came to experiencing angry feelings towards his parents. He feared he would inevitably act upon his rage even when he experienced it solely on a private, internal, emotional basis. Therefore, his feelings could threaten his very survival by pushing him to "bite the hand that feeds him."

Additional layers of emotional complexity emerged, as Abner's participation in treatment deepened. He had become consciously aware of his own tormenting ambivalence. How could he possibly love his parents, if he felt such anger towards them? In Abner's mind, only a monster would not love his own parents. For him, there was no such thing as ambivalence; you either loved someone or hated them. Therefore, Abner avoided creating situations that would intensify his unconscious anger towards his parents. Just like when he was a child, Abner as an adult deftly sidestepped his own needs for their attention. However, he never really renounced this need. Instead, he developed such excruciating pain that even his normally self-absorbed parents were so moved by his suffering that they actually became genuinely solicitous and helpful. Obviously, physical suffering as a covert appeal for emotional responsiveness is not a tenable solution to emotional conflict.

The treatment for psychophysiologic pain syndromes does not require that patients renounce particular feelings. As Abner learned in the course of treatment, feelings are unbidden experiences. We have no control over what we feel, but we can and must exercise control over how we respond to our own feelings. The goal, then, of treatment is to enable the patient to respond to his emotional conflicts more adaptively—by means other than developing pain or other mindbody disorders.

At the outset of treatment, Abner could not recognize his own angry feelings towards his parents because he was not comfortable with such emotional experiences on a private and internal basis.

As Abner understood that angry feelings towards loved ones do not represent an absence of love, he was better able to tolerate the feelings and reflect upon them. Once he was able to maintain his self-esteem while experiencing anger, his pain symptomatology decreased significantly. Abner eventually became completely asymptomatic with respect to his pain symptomatology for a period of five years.

Then Abner's pain recurred in the midst of a family crisis. It was a drama replete with betrayals, recriminations, and anguish usually encountered only in Greek tragedies or soap operas on cable television. His pain was so severe that he required staggering dosages of narcotic analgesics for relief. Even at that, the relief was barely adequate and often short-lived. Nevertheless, Abner never missed a day of work nor even showed up late.

Abner's family insisted he consult the orthopedists who had recommended surgery almost six years before. His family concluded something new must have happened after so long a time without back pain. Abner bowed to their pressures, privately fearing that this episode was different.

Finally, however, Abner concluded that his symptoms could only represent a new outbreak of psychophysiologic back pain despite what doctors and family were telling him.

His realization came from the recognition that he was entirely free of pain during sexual activities (which for him often verged on the acrobatic). A repeat MRI demonstrated no interval change from the original done six years earlier.

In this latest incident, Abner was indeed painfully aware of how angry he felt towards his mother and father for their reckless behavior, which had plunged the entire family into a crisis. Nevertheless, he could not discuss these feelings with his father, whom he believed owned the lion's share of responsibility for the calamity. Abner feared that if he expressed his feelings, it would destroy his father. He observed that the loss of his father would terrify him at least as much as it would sadden him. Abner's dissociated fears of dependency finally emerged. It had always been unsafe for Abner to experience his dependency needs when his parents were so needy and undependable.

The severity of Abner's pain symptomatology alarmed everyone who knew him. He appeared to be a broken man, physically, emotionally, and spiritually. Abner soon came to realize how frightened he was by the magnitude of his rage. He rendered himself harmless by incapacitating himself with excruciating pain. That way he could no longer threaten his father with lethal rage, jeopardizing his own survival. Instead he could indict his father with physical suffering, disarming the father at the same time. No matter how angry his father became in response to his son's veiled accusations, the father could not retaliate with the threat of abandonment when his son was in such dire straits.

As the body language of physical suffering was translated into its emotional substrates, Abner was able to reflect on his fantasies of destructive rage and emotional devastation. Once again, Abner recognized how he protected his father's grandiosity by perpetuating his own sense of dependence.

Despite Abner's prodigious business acumen, he disparaged himself as an impostor, "a boy sent to do a man's job." Abner insured his own survival by not "raining on his father's parade." His natural striving towards independence was weaponized by his own vengeful and competitive feelings towards his father. Therefore, Abner's legitimate ambitions to succeed became entwined with his wish to hurt his father.

As Abner increased his tolerance for his angry and dependent feelings, his pain symptomatology subsided, although not as dramatically as during the first course of treatment. Eventually, Abner was minimally symptomatic on a consistent basis, and he decided to terminate treatment, knowing that more work awaited him.

Critiques of Dr. Sarno's Contributions

Despite Dr. Sarno's success in treating many people who have failed to improve with standard medical and surgical treatments, many physicians and mental health practitioners remain unaware of Dr. Sarno's contributions, or worse, unaware that they are incorrectly informed about his approach to psychophysiologic pain disorders and other mindbody dysfunctions.

Critics of Dr. Sarno point to his role as a powerful transference figure. A transference figure is someone who can revive in us the feelings of near magical intensity we first experienced as children. Mommy kissed our boo-boos and our pain vanished. As adults, physicians whom we endow with fantastic powers, often dispel our fears merely by reassuring us. Transference figures can be menacing, as well as beneficent. How many adults temporarily lose their own senses of competence and autonomy when another person evokes the same feelings they experienced as children being scolded by parents or teachers? In his role as a charismatic transference figure, Dr. Sarno's critics claim, he uses his authority to reassure frightened patients who are desperate to relieve their suffering. However, the same could be said of physicians who sternly warn people about the dire consequences of avoiding surgery. And, analytic clinicians who regard pain symptomatology as an inevitable and immutable effect of aging, injury, or disease—are they not also authoritative transference figures? Rather than disparage clinical improvements as transference cures, it would be more helpful to examine in detail how such intense emotional experiences influence someone's physical suffering. Indeed, if a person's pain symptomatology resolves on the basis of such transference gratifications, does that not convincingly point to the emotional basis for the condition? If only cancer and broken bones were as responsive to the influence of emotional experiences.

Summary

When treatments for musculoskeletal pain are "medicalized," the possibility of approaching these conditions as psychophysiologic disorders is foreclosed. Psychotherapists can readily accept the critical role of emotional conflict in the formation of psychological symptoms such as phobias, obsessions and compulsions, and mood disorders. Unfortunately, this "medicalization" paradigm prevents mental health professionals from recognizing that the same emotional conflicts which lead to psychological symptoms can initiate the development of physical symptoms as well.

Both mental health and medical clinicians unfamiliar with psychophysiologic pain disorders regard the pain as a physiological given, no different from other immutable facts of life. Therefore, the suffering associated with these events cannot be ameliorated by the acquisition of insight.

In order to help the person cope more effectively with these adverse circumstances, the therapist explores how the person reacts to them. The individual's privately held theories or fantasies about being in pain, or losing one's job, for example, are examined to determine if these ideas unnecessarily complicate an already difficult situation. One person might believe these events are punishments for past misdeeds, whereas another individual experiences these situations as permission to shed responsibility without fear of criticism. Therefore, the therapist who is unfamiliar with mindbody disorders misunderstands their pain symptomatology as the proverbial fight looking for a place to happen. Their suffering is an unfortunate "given" which gets recruited by their needs for atonement, or license, for example. These therapists would argue that if Abner and Liam were not in pain, these same psychological needs would seek expression through other life events. In adhering to this treatment model, therapists fail to consider the fact that the psyche may be generating the pain to deflect the person's awareness away from his feelings. Specifically, it is Abner's intolerance of his own angry feelings that initiates a cascade of psychophysiologic events, culminating in excruciating back pain.

Of note, Liam is now an avid, pain-free practitioner of yoga. Abner experiences occasional, minor flare-ups of his pain symptomatology, but remains entirely pain-free for long stretches of time. Neither has resumed treatment. Presumably, if either underwent follow-up medical evaluations, an MRI would reveal the identical findings that prompted doctors initially to recommend surgery.

[2,3] These case histories are from the author's private practice and were provided to Dr. Sarno at his request for use in his book, *The Divided Mind* (ReganBooks, 2006).

PAIN VIGNETTES

Dr. Sarno's clinical formulations of TMS are brought to life and made accessible through case histories. In the next section, I will be presenting clinical vignettes based upon the personality traits and situational triggers Dr. Sarno has identified as key elements in the development of TMS: perfectionism and goodism, anger and self-sacrifice, early childhood trauma, and external events as stressors.

Each of the vignettes I present will focus on one of these key elements. You will recognize, however, that many of these themes recur in each of the histories of these TMS patients. Sometimes a particular theme plays a trivial role in the development of TMS symptomatology; in other cases, it represents the lion's share of the patient's suffering.

The subjects of the vignettes have been selected to portray the most salient dynamic contributing to their pain symptomatology. An appreciation of this dynamic provides the initial access to understanding the patient's unique psychological landscape, which is the first step towards finding pathways to pain relief.

Perfectionism and Goodism

Therese

Therese was a 35-year-old investment banker when she sought treatment for persistent back pain. The pain first developed several weeks after she underwent a caesarean section to deliver twin daughters, two months prematurely. Physicians caring for Therese assumed the pain resulted from the cumulative strain of several months bed rest for a twin pregnancy. Diagnostic studies performed at the time were unremarkable, and doctors assumed these "muscle knots" would work themselves out over time. Therese's pain persisted however, leading her to consult Dr. John Sarno, who recommended individual psychotherapy.

When she began treatment, her daughters were four months old and thriving. No one would have ever suspected Therese had been pregnant, let alone with twins. She had become a supermom, insisting that her house gleam, and that she and her husband sit down to a home-cooked meal every night—all while working sixty hours a week at a high pressure job. As treatment progressed, Therese frequently mentioned a play she had seen. The protagonist was a woman who was not a particularly good cook, kept house poorly, and was considerably overweight. Nevertheless, she was much beloved by the people in her life, especially her rather attractive husband. Therese's reaction was complete disbelief. Although Therese considered the possibility that the play did not necessarily portray life accurately, she was struck by her reaction that she could not even fathom being loved unless she was perfect in every imaginable way.

What especially struck Therese about her reaction was that she could not even fantasize about a state of affairs where she was imperfect but lovable. She remarked, "Even in my imagination, where anything goes, where I'm not constrained by reality, I don't have the internal freedom to imagine being loved when I'm imperfect." She added, "Even if the play doesn't accurately reflect reality, it's still a problem that I'm incapable of even imagining myself in her shoes."

Therese was a much-awaited child. She was born after eight miscarriages, late in her parents' lives. When Therese became a toddler, capable of expressing her own independent wishes, her mother began drinking excessively. Whenever Therese's wishes clashed with her mother's own needs, Therese was berated for being selfish and ungrateful. She compared her relationship with her mother to tiptoeing through a minefield. Therese attempted to recapture the idyllic atmosphere of her earliest childhood by anticipating her mother's needs and synchronizing her behavior to them, thereby avoiding conflict. If she was a perfect daughter, never behaving in any way that would anger her mother, then she would always be safe. This strategy persisted anachronistically into adulthood. Therese never even considered the need to re-evaluate her behavior in light of current realities. She reflexively rolled out her perfectionistic strategies, regardless of their impact on herself and her family.

Perfectionism was a desperate adaptation because it supplied her with the roadmap to tiptoe around minefields. Common sense was the first casualty of her urgent need for emotional safety. When Therese realized that her perfectionistic standards barely improved the quality of her life, she was able to pose the question, "Why am I wasting all this time and energy folding napkins, when it doesn't really contribute to a more pleasant dinnertime for my family?" Over time, she recognized how her perfectionism provided her with only an illusion of emotional safety. Real safety would be achieved once she reappraised the dangers of her childhood in the light of her present day adult resources to cope with them. Perfectionism was a desperate adaptation, which for a long time, had not been a waste of her precious time and energy.

* * *

Perfectionism and goodism are prevalent among individuals suffering from psychophysiologic disorders such as TMS. We are familiar with the term *perfectionism*; Dr. Sarno uses the terms *goodism* and *goodist* in a similar vein. Goodism is perfectionism on a moral plane. In discussing these behaviors, it is important to distinguish between values and psychological defenses. Perfectionism and goodism are defenses aimed at shoring up an individual's sense of vulnerability. Someone perfect is beyond reproach, bullet-proof. Criticism could never wound a perfect person. A perfect person never provokes anger. Indeed, how could a perfect person ever be unloved or abandoned? Perfection is, after all, the ultimate fulfillment of all our dreams.

Adrienne

When Adrienne called to schedule her first appointment, she left a message that dazzled me with her ability to anticipate every inconvenience I might encounter in returning her call. She provided solutions for all the potential obstacles, none of which required any extra effort on my part. Of course, we all appreciate dealing with people who are organized, reliable, and considerate. What underlies Adrienne's goodist behavior is her deeply-held and unexamined conviction that another person could not possibly bear the slightest hardship on her behalf, without regarding her as selfish. The first time Adrienne presented me with an insurance form, rather than fill it out, I only had to sign it. Adrienne consulted all sorts of public records available on the internet to obtain much of the information required by the insurance company, rather than trouble me and risk having me despise her for being so inconsiderate of my valuable time. She barely knew me, but couldn't feel safe enough to expect a routine response from me, such as, "Fine, I'll fill it out and return it to you at our next appointment." Her behavior was not virtuous, it was over the top!

Adrienne, now 54, was the youngest of three children. Her oldest brother was significantly disabled from cerebral palsy, and her older sister exhibited extreme separation anxiety that often required home schooling. Obviously, her parents were under chronic stress from the two older children's special needs.

Whenever Adrienne needed her mother's attention, she was triaged to the back of the line and vilified: "I can't believe how selfish you are. Can't you think of anyone else but yourself? Here I have my hands full with your brother and sister, and you want me to drop everything to look at your coloring book. You are so bad that now I wouldn't look at your goddam coloring book, even if I had the time. Your brother and sister would be so grateful if they were in your shoes that they wouldn't even care about the goddam coloring book." Goodism was essential for Adrienne's survival under such extreme emotional privation. However, what was once a fortress that protected her had now become a prison. Adrienne's goodism didn't make her a better person. It just made her suffer more.

Adrienne, a modern art curator and author of several highly respected works on German expressionism, used to take messages and prepare her shopping list in calligraphy! Everyone values legibility, accuracy, and thoroughness; calligraphy in no way contributes to achieving these goals. Therefore, this extreme example of perfectionism handily captures the differences between a value and a psychological defense. It is easy to see that calligraphy is of absolutely no value when taking messages and making a shopping list. The persistence of such behavior therefore must serve some other purpose.

* * *

In contrast to psychological defenses, values exist independently of emotional rewards and punishments. Parents will discipline a child, even when the child protests, "I hate you mommy," or the equally painful, "I wish you weren't my daddy anymore." As children, we develop our values in the context of emotional rewards and punishments. We learn not to steal in order to win our parents' approval and avoid their censure. To a small child, censure is experienced as "My parents don't love me anymore." As she develops, a child's behavior is motivated more by principle and less by fears of losing parental love. If an adult were lectured by his parents on the folly of paying for goods, the adult would assume his parents' had lost their minds. He would not reconsider his actions and start stealing, just to win his parents' love. Similarly, a patient told me how her teenage son refused to attend Sunday Mass because he no longer believed in God. He proclaimed he was an atheist. However, when he learned that one of the cuter girls in his class regularly attended mass, he found religion again. From his parents' standpoint, he found religion for the wrong reasons. Their son's religious fervor was not based on values, but on his developmentally appropriate need for approval from his peers, especially the very attractive ones.

Patients burdened by their needs to be perfect and saintly at all times are not living according to their own personal code of ethics as much as they are desperately trying to avoid conflict with the important people in their lives. In fact, if goodists could truly believe that conflict was not lethal and that others would indulge their occasional fits of irritability or lack of consideration, they would almost certainly be good people, as opposed to goodists. A patient recovering from surgery, for example, could skip exercise during his two-week convalescence without fearing others will abandon him if his muscle tone decreases or he gains five pounds. When his recovery is complete, he can resume vigorous exercise as an expression of how he values fitness, health, and physical attractiveness.

In *Romeo and Juliet*, Shakespeare observed: "Virtue itself turns vice, being misapplied." With perfectionism and goodism, virtue is misapplied and turns into psychological defense. Perfectionists and goodists are not necessarily closeted slobs, slackers, selfish pigs, or the host of other monstrosities that people fear they will lapse into if they relax their perfectionistic demands. Perfectionism is intrinsically related to an appreciation of quality and rigor in the same way that goodism is fundamentally based upon tenets of decency. During childhood, certain constellations of events teach the child that particular behaviors and attitudes are compulsory, as opposed to highly desirable, and the shift from values to psychological defense occurs. Perfectionism is a compulsive and rigid strategy for bullet-proofing one's psyche. It is not a useful measure of quality control.

Personality Development and Cognitive Development

Both Therese and Adrienne have set themselves apart from the human race. They are perfect and saintly, unblemished by the usual panoply of vices and shortcomings that characterize every other human being.

Are these women morally superior prigs, condescending to everyone within their purview? Or is there something inherently dangerous about being human that impels them into exile for their own protection? Actually, both of these women are gracious to a fault. They are scrupulous in their dealings with people, lest they inadvertently injure or offend someone. Although anything is possible, it would be most surprising to hear someone describe either of these women as sanctimonious.

But what is it about being human that prompts such desperate and drastic measures on their parts? After all, most people make a reasonable go of it, without renouncing their humanity.

To address these issues, it is necessary to take a few steps back and review some basic concepts in personality and cognitive development.

It is well-understood that no event is intrinsically stressful. Stress is a co-creation of an external event and its unique meaning to an individual. Whereas one person experiences retirement as a reprieve, another individual construes the identical situation almost as a death sentence.

How often do friends disagree about someone's attractiveness, or the appeal of a vacation spot or restaurant? Obviously, the pattern of facts remains the same in all of these cases. What differs is each individual's unique set of needs and expectations, which process these facts in very personalized ways. (It is this tendency to react subjectively that provides the basis for psychological tests like the Rorschach, in which people interpret an identical set of inkblots to reveal personality differences.)

This same type of co-creation determines how children metabolize their earliest emotional experiences. All children display temperamental differences from birth. We routinely observe similar traits in animals: skittishness, docility, irritability, and so on. When an angry parent shouts at a skittish child, the child predictably withdraws in fear. A more easygoing child or pet will barely register the event, and soon interacts with the parents or owner as if nothing of significance ever occurred.

Frequently, parents will defend themselves against their children's accusations with, "But your brothers and sisters don't feel that way; that was never a problem for any of them."

Essentially, the parents' disclaimers implicitly recognize that emotional development is not something that is handed down, fully-formed. Instead, it is the final common pathway of multiple, overlapping, and often contradictory influences, including temperament, external events, and even chance factors.

Keeping these features of emotional development in mind, we can better understand why Therese and Adrienne developed such extreme perfectionism and TMS.

For many individuals, conflict is unpleasant, but certainly not lethal. In fact, one can routinely observe cultural differences between groups who tend to avoid confrontation at all costs, and other people who regard disagreement and dissension as an inevitable fact of life, which can be managed, just like any other problem of everyday living. Keep in mind, if emotional reactions were preordained and fixed by their very natures, there would be no cultural or individual variations in the ways people react emotionally to life events.

To both Therese and Adrienne, conflict was equated with the danger of being unlovable. They each feared that if their own mothers even sensed—or worse, experienced—the existence of conflict, they would be perceived as selfish, rejecting, disloyal, or simply, unlovable. And to make matters even worse, their mothers would punish them for these grave defects of character by withdrawing their love from their daughters. What could be more terrifying to a child, whose very existence hinges upon parental caretaking, than the threat of abandonment?

This fear of abandonment, or even annihilation, is poignantly conveyed when chastened children plead in anguish, "I'll be good, I'll be good. I'll do anything you say." Tragically, these pleas are often heard from children who are so abused that the authorities deem it essential for their survival and safety to remove them from their homes. So profound is the child's dependence upon her caretaker, that the fear of abandonment is experienced as a gun to one's head. Who wouldn't sacrifice everything, including all of your own needs, under these circumstances? Even more distressingly, we are talking about children who neither possess nor have access to resources that would allow them to withstand such disruptions in their care.

If a child's natural dependency is experienced by the parents as a life-threatening depletion, and a form of parasitism, then the child sensitive to this aspect of the environment will enshrine self-sufficiency as her salvation. The apparent lack of dependency will be rewarded as much as appeals for help and expressions of need will all be ridiculed as self-indulgent, weak, and selfish—in a word, unlovable.

Obviously, traits such as diplomacy, competence, responsibility, and diligence are highly adaptive, and therefore highly valued. However, in the same way that flowers cannot grow in sand, these traits would never have emerged if Therese and Adrienne had not been born with the potential to develop along these lines, regardless of the early family environment.

Even though these women initially cultivated these behaviors as desperate adaptations, they now exist independently of the circumstances that created them. Therese and Adrienne pride themselves on being responsible, even when slacking off would be inconsequential. Although on first blush this appears to represent an autonomous value system, these behaviors are motivated more by the need for psychological defense than principle.

For example, if someone is tempted to steal an item from an unattended counter in a deli, that person realizes there is a good possibility that his crime will go undetected. He refrains from stealing, however, because it violates his sense of values.

Adrienne and Therese certainly uphold moral principles for all the right reasons. However, neither of them can imagine the world going on if they are rude to a salesclerk, or forget someone's birthday. And although they are genuinely sorry for their occasional human lapses, they are at least as concerned about their lovability, and ultimately, their survival.

These fears persist, unexamined and unmodulated since childhood, even though the two women both have resources to care for themselves, in contrast to their profound helplessness in childhood. Why have they seemingly been unaffected by their adult experience, at least with respect to this area of functioning?

* * *

Let us for a moment take a brief detour into the relationship between cognitive development and personality development.

Emotional development is delimited by cognitive development. An infant whose stroller ends up in the middle of traffic will not experience any terror, because he is too cognitively undeveloped to appreciate such danger. A three-year-old finding himself in that same intersection will scream and cry, because he understands sufficiently the threat he faces.

Similarly, although children gradually develop a sense of time, their cognition remains relatively unnuanced. Any parent can attest to the futility of telling small children, "in an hour" or "later today" or even "tomorrow." All these responses are interpreted by the child as never, ever, ever. They cannot yet take another person's point of view, since they can only understand the world exclusively in terms of their own limited perspective.

These are developmentally normal cognitive responses, not aspects of the child's personality. All children are self-focused, including both many who will grow into considerate, well-related adults, as well as many who will later become fulminant narcissists. So, when a parent drinks alcoholically, the child can only conclude, it must be his fault; he did something wrong to make mommy or daddy act that way.

You can often observe a similar reaction among young children whose parents divorce; the children erroneously believe they are responsible for the breakup of their parents' marriage. They may be at a point developmentally where they are incapable of even considering the possibility that mommy and daddy are separating for reasons entirely unrelated to them and their behavior. The child's immature cognition turns to explanations, such as, "I'm bad, and I'm being punished." After all, reward and punishment are familiar concepts to all young children. The parent's drinking or divorce can therefore only be refracted through the lens of punishment for misbehavior.

If you're bad, it is imperative that you be very, very good—that is, perfect. The undifferentiated nature of young children's cognitive processes doesn't allow for complexity and multiple perspectives. For children, everything is black or white; they are still incapable of perceiving shades of grey.

To a very young child, there can be no such thing as a good girl who did a bad thing. The only possibility given the child's level of cognition is to indict herself as a bad, bad girl.

Because of these cognitive limitations, children cannot be reflective about their own parents' behavior and motives, even as it specifically relates to them. No child, no matter how bright, precocious, or sensitive, could ever conceive of the notion that mommy regards me as a parasite because of her own problems. A child's understanding of the causality of events is always self-referential.

Agency is a psychological concept that describes a person's sense of his own ability to influence and control the circumstances of his life. Very young children often experience themselves as possessing limitless power to affect the circumstances of their lives. Although the child's exalted sense of agency is cognitively determined, this inordinate sense of responsibility and power shapes the child's emotional experiences as well.

Children exhibit magical thinking—that is, they believe that wishing makes something so. Their very own thoughts are all-powerful. Although omnipotence is very reassuring to the helpless, dependent child, this same power can be terrifying. When a child stamps his feet in protest while shouting, "You're not my mommy (or daddy) anymore," the child simultaneously fears he may have destroyed his only source of sustenance, because his wishes are so powerfully destructive.

If the parent responds spitefully with, "Well I don't want you to be my little girl anymore," then the child's worst fears materialize. The child has now learned that thoughts and feelings—private, internal, emotional experiences—are potential sources of danger that could jeopardize relationships essential for his survival.

* * *

Applying this understanding of personality vs. cognitive development to Therese's and Adrienne's situations, we can now appreciate the impossibility for either of them accurately to place their mothers' behaviors in context.

They were selfish, disloyal, and unloving—always, and to everyone they would ever meet. A young child's crude cognition could never generate an alternative, such as, "Mother may disapprove, but others will like me." These young girls are essentially backed into corners, because they cannot envision a way out of these emotional straits.

In this context perfection becomes a magical amulet. It can disarm people and insure the child's safety. Perfectionism has all the characteristics that immature cognition can recognize and grab hold of. Perfectionism is undifferentiated—that is, it is all or nothing.

Perfectionism does not take into account anyone else's perspective. By its very nature, perfectionism is devoid of perspective. Perfectionism actually disintegrates when perspective can be achieved. The question remains unanswered, however, as to why Therese and Adrienne have failed to achieve perspective with respect to their perfectionistic demands.

There is a story that may help shed light on the dynamic at play here. During the 1960s, the Philippine government was clearing the jungles as part of a land-development and modernization project. They discovered a Japanese soldier hiding in the jungle. To everyone's amazement, he was entirely unaware that World War II had ended some 20 years before.

After their initial shock, the developers and the soldier could readily reconstruct and apprehend his dilemma. If the war was still being waged, the soldier remained safer hidden in the jungle. On the other hand, if the war was over, he was hiding in vain. In order to find out if the war was still raging, however, he would have to risk his safety. For the soldier, safety was paramount.

Similarly, it is possible that either Therese or Adrienne could have tested the waters at a later point in their lives. Perhaps other people were not as critical and fragile as their own mothers had been? Yet, what if that wasn't the case? They felt they couldn't chance it, at least not until the physical pain of TMS presented another, though different kind of danger.

* * *

Therese then became symptomatic as she tried to juggle her career along with her perfectionistic demands for housekeeping and parenting. Therese was baffled as to why these demands were so non-negotiable in her own mind.

Her husband could have cared less if the napkins were folded. He preferred Chinese take-out and pizza to home-cooked meals exquisitely presented. If anything, he felt somewhat put out by her elaborate preparations. He was more apt to regard her behavior as "just plain nuts" as opposed to admirable. While he appreciated a clean and orderly home, he was not intolerant of occasional messes and clutter. He repeatedly offered to hire as much household help as Therese felt she needed, rather than witness her self-flagellation for minor lapses in housekeeping.

And with me, Adrienne did not score extra points when she gave me her completed insurance form requiring only my signature. I wasn't impressed with her unusual level of consideration for others. I was distressed by how extreme her behavior was, as well as moved by how fearful she must be that she couldn't automatically assume I would be appropriately responsive and more than willing to both complete and sign the form for her.

If I had reacted critically to Adrienne for "presumptuously" expecting me to complete an insurance form, Adrienne would not have immediately regarded my behavior as inappropriate.

Similarly, had Therese's husband, mother, or in-laws commented about a mess or an accumulation of dust, it is doubtful that she would be able to recognize their impertinence and defend herself with conviction.

The very loss of perspective, which initiates perfectionism, also maintains it, creating the impression that one is impervious to outside influences. In the same way it's challenging to maintain grace under pressure, it's at least as difficult to maintain perspective when they're shooting bullets at your feet, especially when you can't even consider the possibility that they're shooting blanks or BBs, not weapons of mass destruction. Or, that you're not completely vulnerable. Adults can wear bullet-proof vests, or dodge the bullet and seek shelter. They can also call the police. Adults are aware of a range of possibilities; there are flesh wounds, fender benders, wrecks, and mortal wounds. Children, on the other hand, are a captive audience and can only imagine the worst. Despite their impressive achievements as adults, aspects of both Therese's and Adrienne's personalities were still frozen in time and unreachable to the present. They experienced themselves as frightened children instead of competent adults. They were still unable to recognize and utilize their adult resources to reappraise the original dangers that drove them into hiding in their own version of the Philippine jungle, namely perfectionism.

No matter how saintly anyone could possibly be, it is impossible not to experience rage towards powerful figures who blackmail you into submission. Parents of teenagers will immediately recognize how their children are often angry at them simply because their children resent their own sense of enforced dependence. Most people with TMS are unaware of experiencing such complicated feelings of anger and need. In fact, consciously experiencing such emotional reactions would challenge their aspirations to sainthood. It is important to emphasize that feeling anger is not the same as expressing anger. Feelings are private, internal, emotional experiences. Emotional expressions are actions. We will discuss later how the failure to distinguish reliably between feelings and actions contributes to the development of TMS. For either Therese or Adrienne to express anger towards their parents would be tantamount to "biting the hand that fed them." Simply, starvation is even worse than subsistence. When Therese and Adrienne behave perfectly, they can still control (that is to say, assure) their safety. But if they express anger, then they have fallen from grace. You cannot be perfect if you express anger. And you certainly can't be perfect if your behavior provokes anger, criticism, or censure. Therefore, even if you express anger appropriately, and even if that expression of anger is completely justified, all bets are off. You're officially now on your own; you've been abandoned by the only people who could sustain you. This doomsday scenario is the script that Therese, Adrienne, and other perfectionists follow.

Except in cases of extreme depravity, when children misbehave, their parents do not starve them, or place them in foster care, or deposit them on the nearest church doorstep. No doubt there were many instances when Adrienne and Therese misbehaved, given the nature of children, and the duration of childhood. Although their parents reacted inappropriately at times, it is also true that their parents responded empathically to them as well. Nevertheless, neither Therese nor Adrienne could utilize these experiences as children, to re-evaluate the mandates for their perfectionism.

Self-esteem is the feeling of positive or negative regard about oneself which is derived from self-evaluation. Self-esteem is inevitably inadequate when perfection is the standard of acceptability. Therese and Adrienne always experienced themselves as the proverbial beggars, who can never be choosers. They have always been so preoccupied with the urgency of surviving, that they can't reflect on the range of experiences that were an everyday part of their lives. For them, there were only two options: dead or alive. You can't reflect on a range of experiences when the only two choices are black and white. That loss of perspective reinforces the perfectionism. Therefore, they are unable to utilize the notion of a track record, which is predicated upon the ability to develop perspective. Despite repeated opportunities in their childhoods and adult lives to observe parents and other important figures behaving selfishly or generously, for example, they can never conclude that someone is basically good, but screwed up today. And, of course, the same applies to them as well. When perfectionism sets the standards for self-evaluation, the results can only be cast in all-or-nothing terms. Their limited view of the world essentially filters out precisely the information that would challenge the need to maintain perfectionism. Humans cannot see ultraviolet or infrared rays, even though they exist everywhere. Similarly, perfectionism operates like a set of blinders that limits the person's field of vision, or perspective.

Anger and Self-Sacrifice

Anger is the mortal enemy of perfectionism. Children's immature cognition allows them to believe that they are transparent to adults. Therefore, just quietly thinking critical thoughts, or privately feeling anger towards powerful parental figures will be objectionable. Expressing anger is absolutely incompatible with perfection. Perfection can only work as a winning strategy in the complete absence of anger. So, what if the firewall between feeling and acting isn't failsafe—that is, perfectly secure? The only option is to bolster your petition for canonization. Although mere mortals feel resentment when they are not taken care of, perfectionists, aspiring to be true saints, castigate themselves for their pettiness and self-centeredness whenever they experience human emotions such as resentment, jealousy, and desire. They appear happily to renounce their own needs and devote themselves to caring for others. However, these apparent sacrifices are actually grudging concessions made only to avoid conflict. Rarely does the person with TMS have conscious awareness of the anguished connection between selflessness and anger. If one has no needs of his own, then there is no basis for conflict, anger, disappointment, frustration, or fears of being burdensome. Who couldn't love such a selfless child, or adult?

Unfortunately, this winning strategy fails to take into account that no one can completely escape his or her humanity. The only exemption from the human race is death. Furthermore, true saints do experience anger, doubt, lust, jealousy, even vengefulness. What distinguishes saints from ordinary men and women is how they deal with these feelings, not the mistaken notion that they are fundamentally incapable of experiencing them.

So if anger can defeat perfectionism, what's a poor saint like Therese or Adrienne or other people with TMS to do? The simple answer is to develop TMS. It is important to clarify and emphasize that the development of TMS is never a conscious choice. No one wakes up in the morning and says to himself, "Today I will develop TMS," in the same way someone might decide to put on a red sweater, or a black pleated skirt, or order a toasted bagel for breakfast.

We need to debunk the overly simplistic idea that TMS is self-inflicted. If someone is driving along a ribbon of coastal highway when the car loses traction with the road, it is essential for that driver's survival to try and ram the car into the embankment, rather than risk certain death or profound disability by allowing the car to plunge into the ocean. Can we accurately characterize injuries as self-inflicted, when the driver sustains multiple fractures, a ruptured spleen, and punctured lungs by intentionally ramming into the embankment to avoid something far worse? These injuries reflect a successful adaptation to desperate circumstances. Similarly, when someone develops TMS, it too is a successful adaptation to the desperate circumstances of fearing for your safety. Like the car crash, where no one would question the potential for catastrophe, we must understand why the patient with TMS feels so imperiled that developing pain is unconsciously the lesser of two or more evils.

Pain is such a compelling distraction that nothing can successfully compete for someone's awareness when they are struggling to endure pain. Emotions are disguised as physical suffering. If you don't know you're angry because it's disguised, then you can honestly claim you're not angry. There is no need to fear the eruption of anger, because there is no anger. And just in case a little bit of anger leaks out, pain punishes the infraction. Pain tortures everyone who cares about the TMS patient, while insulating the patient from other people's anger and resentment. After all, who can blame someone who is suffering? Only a monster would feel anger toward someone in such a piteous state. Suffering disarms, muzzles, and whips into shape anyone who even dares to think or express a critical thought or feeling.

TMS turns the tables: A person with TMS can now express anger safely without jeopardizing the person's security. The person's pain repackages and camouflages anger. Neither the individual nor those around him know he's angry—he's just suffering. Pain provides a legitimate excuse to relax one's perfectionistic demands without incurring a penalty. Pain also validates an individual's entitlement to caretaking, while protecting him from his own and others' accusations of selfishness. TMS is the psyche's versatile solution to conflicts over anger and dependency—except for the fact that it is extremely painful and debilitating.

Since perfectionism, goodism, and TMS all ultimately fail to eliminate emotional and physical suffering, the only solution is for the TMS patient to figure out how to rejoin the human race, without feeling constantly endangered. Throughout this book, we will be following the different paths patients have blazed for themselves as they recovered from TMS.

Peter

Peter was a 40-year-old architect and father of four young children. His two oldest were stepchildren from his wife's brief first marriage, whom he adopted.

When Peter would take the children to the county fair during summer vacation, they bickered constantly in the backseat of the minivan. Even though Peter intellectually recognized that children squabble in the backseats of cars, he was appalled and frightened when he found himself fantasizing about getting out of the car and leaving his kids by the side of the road to fend for themselves.

He automatically assumed that no loving father could ever think of such a thing. A good father can only have loving feelings towards his children, no matter how exasperatingly and ungratefully they behaved. Peter concluded he must be a despicable person. Deeply ashamed of what he considered to be his grave shortcomings, he was afraid that people would shun him if they discovered the true nature of his character. He even feared that his wife would leave him and take the children. Though he was a devoted parent, his recognition of this was of no consolation. In fact, Peter piled on further self-reproaches: Now he was a hypocrite in addition to being a monster.

To make matters worse, Peter's wife, whom he often described as a clone of Bree Van de Kamp from *Desperate Housewives*, prided herself on how much she loved being a mother, so much so that the children never even got on her nerves.

Obviously, if she could do it, then it had to be possible for Peter to feel that perfect love for one's own children. At that point, Peter could not even consider that "the lady," in this case his wife, "doth protest too much." He was incapable of even considering that his wife's claims of "perfect love" represented her own psychological defenses against conflict, and not a true indication of her sterling character. By comparison, Peter's failure to love his children unambivalently was tantamount to an unforgivable mortal sin.

Actually, Peter didn't realize he was normal. Ambivalence characterizes all significant relationships. The presence of ambivalence merely confirms a person's humanity. However, Peter's reaction was unusual because he was consciously aware of experiencing negative feelings, in contrast to many people with TMS.

It is important to understand how someone experiences his or her own ambivalence, as well as how the person handles these feelings. For many people like Peter, feelings are understood to operate according to the rules of algebra—that is, a positive feeling cancels out a negative one. They have an implicit but mistaken belief that feelings conform to linear scientific models, whereas feelings are actually non-rational. (I am deliberately avoiding the word *irrational* because it connotes insanity and loss of control.) By non-rational, I mean nonlinear, like poetry or humor, as opposed to algebra and physics, which are both logical and systematic.

Anger and love often co-exist, in anguish or acceptance. Anger does not cancel out love, nor vice versa—except in the minds of insistent goodists whose sense of moral perfectionism demands a purity of heart for defensive purposes.

Often when people recognize their ambivalence, they react with horror. To them, ambivalence questions the authenticity, depth, and durability of their feelings. Maybe my love isn't true, perhaps my love isn't strong enough, or might I be fickle and confused?

Of course, someone might be all of those things, but none of that means that ambivalent love isn't profound, long-lasting, and real. For many people, however, the recognition of ambivalent feelings is unbearable, because it poses a direct threat to the integrity of their self-image.

In Honolulu, there is a statue commemorating General Douglas MacArthur. The accompanying plaque reads: "Bravery is not the absence of fear, but the ability to bear it." Similarly, theologians of all stripes argue that faith is not the absence of doubt, but the ability to persist in one's beliefs despite it. Indeed, if there were no doubt, why would there ever be a need for faith?

Many people with TMS attempt to purify their ambivalence by banishing negative emotions from their awareness. Instead of a jumble of conflicting feelings, they are now relieved of their guilt feelings, experiencing only uncomplicated love towards the powerful figures in their lives. If the patient can successfully capture and contain his anger, then he can achieve a perfected state of non-ambivalence.

The Lethality of Anger

For Peter and many people suffering with TMS, anger threatens to completely and permanently destroy relationships deemed essential to their survival. Peter's world is painted only in black or white; there is no color or shades of gray in his emotional landscape. For them, anger is never temporary or trifling; it never exists along a continuum of feeling. It is always, and can only be, lethal.

Indifference is actually the opposite of love, but for people with TMS, anger equals the threat of unlovability. Peter was unable to dispel his feelings of shame and self-loathing, even when he reminded himself of how devoted he was to his children. As with Therese and Adrienne, Peter's internal experience could not be modulated by present day facts. Here, again, we are led to ask: How has Peter been able to maintain his morbid fears about anger's deadly power, when a preponderance of his experiences contradict those fears?

Peter lost perspective a long time ago. The primitive equation that anger is bad, love is good, and never the twain shall meet, arose out of his earliest experiences. Then it overdetermined his adult development.

Because he was so focused on his survival—which is to say, maintaining his lovability—he was unable to see the evidence which would have put his fears into perspective.

If you cannot register the information from these new experiences, then you can't integrate it and utilize it in the future. If you can avoid an awareness of the complexity of your own emotional experiences, however, you can escape the torments of ambivalence. Unfortunately, in this process, he let his self-reminders about his loving connections to his children just pass through him like a sieve.

Peter is no longer ambivalent. Instead, he is completely consumed with self-loathing for his angry feelings. If only his moral superiority could prevail over his anger, all would be right in the world.

Joyce McDougall (1989), the French psychoanalyst who has written extensively about mindbody disorders, has characterized "symptoms as attempts at self-care." When all other options have been exhausted, TMS can become a form of self-care. Perfectionism here perpetuates the vicious cycle of anger and self-sacrifice. Only when Peter's pain became worse than his fears of his own anger did he risk confronting his true lovability.

Peter described the atmosphere of his early childhood by referring to his father's two favorite sayings: "You're either with me, or against me," and "Blood is thicker than water." Peter, his two sisters and brother, and his mother were all expected to display unwavering respect towards the head of the household, "no questions asked, period, case closed."

Despite his dogmatic nature, Peter's father was devoted to his family. A tireless worker, he routinely signed up for extra shifts at the textile plant where he worked as a foreman, in order to provide his family with every advantage, including education at prestigious universities.

When Peter entered adolescence, he naturally began to separate from his family. His father would tolerate occasional curfew violations while shrugging his shoulders and muttering philosophically, "Boys will be boys."

As an inquisitive teenager, Peter often challenged his father's political beliefs and religious values. At these times, his father would become apoplectic and threatened to disown his son and throw Peter out of the house for his disloyalty and ingratitude. Sadly, Peter's father's connection to his son was severed by conflict. For Peter's father, independence, insubordination, disloyalty, rejection, and betrayal were all rolled up together in the same emotional ball of wax. In order to restore the tie to his father, Peter would first plead for his father's forgiveness. Before his father would finally relent, Peter had to recant his divergent views and apologize for his betrayal.

Peter's internal experience was the operational definition of ambivalence; he wanted both to please and destroy his father at the same time. His sense of self could not encompass the full range of his feelings without fearing he would disintegrate. Bitter resentment towards his father's dictatorial exercise of power disrupted Peter's sense of being a loving and loyal son. On the other hand, whenever Peter considered how his father championed his son's advanced professional training, rather than feeling soothed by the memory, Peter reviled himself as weak and spineless. Now tenderness towards his father threatened to undermine his sense of himself as a strong and resolute man. Peter's self-cohesion could not withstand this maelstrom of conflicting feelings. By drastically truncating his access to these unruly feelings, Peter could enforce a fragile emotional cease-fire.

When Peter's emotional rigidity could no longer protect his brittle self-esteem from shattering, he developed TMS. In his treatment, Peter learned that feelings were private emotional experiences, not measures of morality. This knowledge emboldened Peter to explore the complexity of his inner life. Previously, the only feelings available to him were anger and fear of abandonment. Consequently, his self-experience was limited to regarding himself exclusively as bad, weak, and hypocritical. Under these conditions, his feelings are disproportionately intense because they are not modulated by a wider range of experiences. By elaborating the full context in which his feelings existed, Peter was able to develop perspective. Now his resentment towards his children no longer defined him; it represented just one aspect of his entire being. Instead of feeling like a bad father and a fraud, Peter was now able to experience himself as a loving father who would occasionally feel angry towards his children. His angry feelings were no longer intolerable because he could maintain his self-esteem while experiencing them fully. As Peter consolidated his ability to experience ambivalence and psychological integrity simultaneously, his TMS gradually subsided.

Childhood Experience

Antoinette

When Antoinette, a 40-year-old Pilates instructor, entered treatment for debilitating back pain, her son had just turned two. Antoinette's pain had begun almost three years before. She had undergone disc surgery without benefit. She was desperate, fearing she was running out of options. She was also becoming addicted to the narcotics prescribed by her physicians to control her excruciating pain.

Antoinette's son was conceived through in-vitro fertilization and her partner of 11 years carried the pregnancy to term. Obviously, such a conception does not occur accidentally. Nevertheless, once her partner's pregnancy was confirmed, Antoinette's mood soured. Fearing she would lose her partner's exclusive attention, she became jealous of their unborn child. Once their son was born, she experienced her partner's appropriate devotion to their son's needs as abandonment. She grew increasingly resentful of both her partner and son. Antoinette not only felt guilty and ashamed of these feelings, but her relationship with both her partner and son became increasingly strained. In retrospect, Antoinette realized her back pain first developed as she and her partner were undergoing fertility treatments in preparation for the in-vitro fertilization.

Antoinette is the oldest of three children; her sister is two years younger and her brother is almost six years younger than her. When her brother was born, Antoinette, who was almost six, felt as if the world had come to an end. Growing up, Antoinette was outshone by her younger brother, who was both a better athlete and student. Moreover, Antoinette's intense personality clashed with her mother's emotional volatility, in contrast to her brother's more easygoing temperament, which always seemed to soothe the mother. So when Antoinette's son was born, it was déjà vu. A man once again stole the love of her life away from her. The birth of Antoinette's son reawakened long-buried, unresolved feelings surrounding her brother's birth. Antoinette was now reacting to her son as though the boy was her rival.

In an odd twist, TMS came to the rescue. When debilitating pain was insufficient to distract Antoinette from her jealous hatred of her son, the staggering doses of narcotics offered an additional level of protection by clouding Antoinette's consciousness. Furthermore, the entire household re-oriented itself around Antoinette and her needs. She was now the focus of everyone's attention and concern. Her rightful place had been restored. The challenge that we faced in treatment was how Antoinette could reconfigure her childhood relationships to feelings of competence, need, independence, and isolation without developing new or recurrent psychophysiologic symptoms.

* * *

Childhood experiences shape our personalities, and our subsequent experiences are refracted through this developing character structure. A personality that is organized so that it interprets emotional closeness as vulnerability will be unable to derive any comfort from that closeness. Similarly, a personality that was forged in a home where helplessness was confused with lovability will never enjoy the thrill of independence and achievement. In fact, success will threaten and frighten such an individual.

Every personality organization has its own unique fault lines, areas of increased sensitivity and vulnerability to stress, just like the fault lines in the earth's crust. When the earth's fault lines are stressed by seismic events, the earth quakes. When we experience stress along our emotional fault lines, we are much more likely to develop emotional distress and psychophysiologic conditions.

The case of Antoinette, along with the cases of Nicholas and Karl which follow, demonstrate how present day events can tear open the scabs from previously healed wounds and contribute to the development of TMS.

Unresolved feelings are like ghosts that come back to haunt us. There are two questions we must examine in order to understand Antoinette's pain symptomatology more thoroughly. First, why were her feelings of sibling rivalry unresolved, whereas other disappointing, wounding, or even shameful experiences from her past were clearly resolved?

During her childhood, Antoinette developed intensely rivalrous feelings towards her brother. She dreamed about having front row seats to her brother's failure and public humiliation. Feeling utterly worthless, Antoinette was consumed with rage. She was furious with both of her parents for inflicting painful feelings of inferiority on her by favoring her brother. But her fury morphed into self-reproach: How could anyone as inadequate as Antoinette even have the audacity to be angry and critical of other people?

In her mind, Antoinette's parents were already disappointed with her for her lackluster academic performance and disobedience. If they ever found out that she harbored such vengeful feelings toward her own brother, they would have no choice but to disown her. No daughter of theirs could possibly be that selfish and resentful.

For Antoinette, as for many other individuals with TMS, a do-or-die conflict between anger and lovability sets the stage for the future development of TMS.

For Antoinette, her destructive wishes toward her brother

were intolerable. For her, such feelings were *prima facie* evidence of her worthlessness. She was unable to recognize her feelings simply as feelings. The mere existence of these negative feelings confirmed her defective nature and justified in her own mind her fears of rejection by her family. Antoinette could not maintain positive self-esteem so long as she experienced these feelings, even on a private, internal, emotional basis. Her anger became unbearable because it simultaneously threatened both her self-esteem and sense of self-cohesion.

Feelings can be resolved only when the individual can meaningfully interact with them. One can only reflect upon feelings which are consciously recognized as a part of oneself. Losses can then be mourned, preparing the way for new experiences.

Unresolved feelings represent losses that have been denied, and therefore unmourned. Resolved feelings can rest in peace, having been integrated into the totality of the individual's experiences. Since unresolved feelings remain in a state of perpetual non-integration, they lurk along the sidelines, haunting us like ghosts who return to settle scores and attend to unfinished business. When people come to terms with their feelings, they are then capable of moving on or letting go.

Experiencing the Past in a New Way

To understand more completely Antoinette's dilemma, let's briefly digress to examine in detail the fate of both resolved and unresolved feelings. The following example describes the transition from adolescence into adulthood and its vicissitudes. This struggle, in all of its permutations, is recognizable to everyone. Although conflicts around independence and dependence, and responsibility and freedom, are most salient during this developmental phase, the same dynamics characterize the resolution of all ambivalent feelings, especially conflicts over love and anger.

Mark Twain observed, "When I was nineteen, I thought my father was the dumbest man in the world. Now that I'm twenty, I'm amazed at how much he's learned in one year." Obviously, the basis for making either of these observations is the same in both cases. The lens through which the young man sees the world is the only factor that has changed. The past is now experienced in a new and different way. Through maturation, the young man resolves the typical adolescent conflicts over dependency and autonomy. He is no longer holding on to such feelings as, "You're controlling me," or "You're treating me like a child," or "You just don't want to see me have any fun." Instead, these feelings are supplanted by a new experience of himself that can embrace both consideration of others along with independence. Accommodation to others, which was previously regarded as a humiliating loss of freedom, is no longer experienced as defeat or submission. The very same past, which previously oppressed them, is now experienced in a new way. Life lessons are now integrated into the individual's psyche, where they have been transformed from humiliating reminders of adolescent powerlessness into mature, adult resources.

People exhibiting immaturity or arrested development exemplify what we call a "Peter Pan Syndrome." These individuals never resolve conflicts over separation and individuation. They are tyrannized by their pasts, and the past persists indefinitely into their present and future. These people can never acknowledge or come to terms with their yearning to be indulged and exempt from all responsibility. For them, even admitting such wishes is too mortifying to endure. It undermines the credibility of their insistence upon complete freedom, which routinely gets confused with independence in the minds of adolescents. Therefore, there is no possibility to achieve a truce with themselves and their parental overlords when they are so completely out of touch with their feelings. Adults reconcile themselves to the lamentable fact that there is no such thing as unlimited freedom. Adults can recognize the limits to freedom without experiencing a crushing loss of self-esteem. They can mourn their losses and move on, without the self-reproaches that unlimited freedom would be available if they were less a sell-out and more courageous. The adult possesses the resources to obtain both caretaking and freedom. For the Peter and Petra Pans of the world, the unresolved longing for complete freedom prevents the past from being laid to rest. Although it's impossible to dispute the past is the past, the past affects the present in different ways, whether it's resolved or unresolved. Memories provide a link to the past, which serves as a valuable resource for dealing with the demands and challenges of the present and the future. Ghosts, on the other hand, represent the inescapable past.

* * *

With respect to the effects of resolved and unresolved feelings on an individual's psychological makeup and functioning, it becomes apparent how Antoinette's disavowal of her feelings certainly predisposed her to developing TMS. Yet why didn't she develop a drinking problem, or a depression, or some kind of other exclusively psychological disorder? Even if we invoke the concept of somatic compliance—that the psyche exploits a constitutional physical vulnerability—it still doesn't explain why the body becomes the preferred mode for expressing feelings and emotional distress.

Antoinette's feelings terrified her. They revealed her base nature and threatened to out her to her family as a despicable individual masquerading as a good person. If a monster and a fraud, she is undeserving of love and caring. Furthermore, she didn't know how to handle her feelings except to stifle them or impulsively express them. Either choice would have been disastrous.

The brother was especially prized for his agreeable nature, whereas Antoinette was criticized sharply for making waves. Consequently, whenever Antoinette expressed feelings, she experienced herself as defective and in danger of rejection. Antoinette sought refuge from emotional disruption by being out of touch with her feelings. Once Antoinette excluded her painful feelings from awareness, they were cut off from the influences that fostered her maturation in other areas. Unfortunately, her self-protection was the very thing that stunted Antoinette's emotional development, leaving her even more vulnerable to the uncontrolled force of her emotions.

For Antoinette, back pain indicated the existence of a fixable, structural problem, in contrast to emotional pain, which called into question her very being. She felt more in control with her body than with her unwieldy feelings. Therefore, physical suffering frightened her less than emotional anguish. Not surprisingly, Antoinette gravitated to personal training as a career, where she excelled professionally. When Antoinette's back hurt, she could get extra rest or bend from her knees. And yet, unsuccessful back surgery undermined her belief in the structural etiology of her back pain. Now, Antoinette's body was a battlefield instead of a refuge from her terrifying feelings.

During treatment, Antoinette gradually verbalized her fear that, as a parent, she was no longer eligible for dependent care. Previously, she expressed this same fear through body language. She was so incapacitated by back pain that she required almost the same level of caretaking as her infant son. As she continued to put her feelings into words, she experienced them as less chaotic and more differentiated. In revisiting her childhood experiences, she was able to view her emotional turbulence through the light of present day realities. Her mature understanding that dependency was neither inherently despicable nor absolute, modulated the intensity of the primitive fears which first emerged during her childhood. Similarly, she was able to revise her previously unrecognized fears that independence always and automatically resulted in isolation and the permanent and complete loss of dependent care. Antoinette also integrated this newly acquired self-knowledge into her sense of self. Now her anger was regarded as a private, internal, emotional experience, which no longer defined her as a monster. Instead, it was merely one aspect of her complex inner world. Antoinette eventually realized that the same strategy that insulated her from emotional pain also deprived her of the opportunity to master her feelings and avoid developing TMS.

The Reawakening of Childhood Trauma

Nicholas

Nicholas, a 60-year-old retired pianist, initially came to treatment for persistent low back pain, which radiated down both of his legs. His pain symptomatology gradually resolved as he identified his angry feelings toward Maria, his wife of almost 25 years. At the beginning of treatment, Nicholas feared that any evidence of angry feelings doomed his relationship. It was mandatory that Nicholas banish such experiences from his conscious mind. To Nicholas, it was preferable, and consequently easier, to experience himself as someone debilitated by chronic pain, than to entertain the possibility that he was angry at Maria.

After Nicholas' pain symptomatology resolved, he decided to continue on in treatment to address more thoroughly his people-pleasing behaviors. Not only did his fears of conflict adversely affect his relationship with Maria, but they also had limited his career opportunities when he was younger.

At one point in the treatment, Nicholas and Maria's cherished dog suddenly became ill when a canine virus swept through New York. Although the dog became listless and emaciated, the veterinarian had assured them the dog was expected to survive and ultimately regain her health. Nevertheless, Nicholas became preoccupied with the dog's undernourished appearance, even though she was gradually regaining the weight she had lost. He became obsessed with every morsel of food she ate and every morsel of food she turned down. At this same time, Nicholas re-experienced the back and sciatic pain that hadn't plagued him in almost three years. Nicholas was especially baffled by his recurrent pain, because he could see their dog was improving slowly.

As we explored his emotional reactions, Nicholas brought up memories of the deaths of his father and younger sister when he was ten. We had discussed these tragic losses many times during the course of his treatment.

His father died of leukemia and his sister died several days later from cystic fibrosis. For as long as Nicholas could remember, his family was constantly maintaining bedside vigils for his father and sister, who both required frequent and prolonged hospitalizations.

This time when we discussed their illnesses, Nicholas recalled vividly how skeletal they both appeared weeks before their deaths. In fact, both of them often refused food, despite his mother's anguished pleading and the efforts of relatives to tempt them with luscious homemade desserts and favorite foods. Nicholas immediately realized how his preoccupation with his dog's weight and nutritional intake paralleled the helpless terror he must have experienced watching his father and sister die before his eyes. His dog's illness had "ripped off the scabs" from these incompletely healed emotional wounds. The pain resurfaced to protect him from more direct contact with those raw and overpowering feelings. Because he was in treatment, however, Nicholas responded to his pain symptomatology as a signal to guide his introspection, not as evidence of a new physical disorder. Nicholas' pain symptomatology slowly improved as he belatedly mourned these tragic losses.

As Nicholas' father and sister were dying, his mother was overwhelmed by her own grief and preoccupied by her fears for the future. Consequently, she was unavailable to Nicholas, who relatively speaking could at least fend for himself. His extended family, consisting of eight aunts and his maternal grandmother, all naïvely tried to protect Nicholas by discouraging any talk about the tragedies surrounding him.

Their misguided behavior unfortunately dovetailed with a sense of "every man for himself" that dominated the atmosphere at home. Nicholas was essentially left to cope with the impending loss of his sister and father all by himself. Equipped with only the resources of a 10-year-old boy, he was overwhelmed without even realizing it. Nicholas was traumatized, helpless to comprehend fully the impact of these deaths and the ensuing disruption to his family's stability. The magnitude of this tragedy nearly erased his already limited ability to cope without adult assistance. He was shut down, barely functioning on automatic pilot. Since no adults were available to help him make sense of his emotional reactions to this catastrophe, in desperation his psyche hurled these events into a jury-rigged, interior black box to be processed at a later date when the coast was clear.

This experience remained there for many years as an undigested, disorganized, and wordless blob of emotions. The sight of Nicholas' dog's emaciated appearance unleashed a tsunami of emotion, which Nicholas experienced as pain because the original loss had never been put into words. When feelings cannot be organized around thoughts and put into words, they cannot be understood as meaningful. Feelings without meaning can never be mastered, and instead are often experienced by the body as painful physical sensations. For Nicholas, the recurrent pain was like a flashback that directed us to that wordless state of terror he first experienced as a 10-year-old boy.

Karl

Karl Heinz was an almost 40-year-old advertising executive when he sought treatment for back pain that had tyrannized his life since turning 30. A self-described free spirit, Karl especially relished shocking others with his unconventional attitudes and nontraditional lifestyle. When he began treatment, Karl had been living with Kevin for almost 15 years. They were raising Kevin's three daughters from his two previous marriages. Karl professed revulsion at the idea of marriage, which had recently become an option for same-sex couples. This was fortunate because Kevin had vowed never to marry again after two failed marriages and an especially bruising second divorce.

Around the time his back pain began, Karl recalled a particularly rancorous encounter with Kevin's second wife. Against medical advice, the ex-wife had just checked herself out of a psychiatric hospital, where she had been undergoing treatment for recurrent manic episodes. During an exchange over Kevin's youngest daughter's difficulties adjusting to middle school, the ex-wife lashed out at Karl, screaming, "Kevin married two women, but he won't marry you. He doesn't love you enough to marry you. And he still loves me!" Karl brushed aside these cruel remarks as the baseless rantings of an embittered and disturbed woman.

He reminded himself how he belittled the institution of marriage as nothing more than a throwback to medieval times.

Nevertheless, he realized that he felt wounded by the ex-wife's taunts. Karl recalled that although he felt secure in Kevin's love for him, at least most of the time, he did resent that Kevin never seemed to defend him against his ex-wife's attacks. He always explained away his tolerance of his ex-wife's outbursts, saying she was severely mentally ill, one of the chief reasons he divorced her in the first place. Although his reasoning made sense to Karl, somehow Kevin's explanations were never completely satisfying.

Karl Heinz, who preferred to be called Karl, related how his family moved from a small town outside of Munich, Germany when he was 3½ to an even smaller town in the Pacific Northwest for his father's job. He moved again as he was entering second grade, this time to New York City. He felt unable to penetrate the cliques that others had already formed. Karl was overweight at the time and looked like a "mini-lumberjack." While the students didn't ridicule him, they never invited him to join them. His parents never "defended" him by intervening on his behalf. They never discussed Karl's social problems with his teacher. They never reached out to the parents of his classmates. They also never enrolled him in group activities where he would have additional opportunities to interact with his peers and begin to develop friendships.

Instead, his parents encouraged his participation in more solitary activities like skateboarding and martial arts. Karl could only make sense of what he was experiencing as a seven-year-old. He automatically assumed he was unworthy and unlovable. It never could have occurred to him at his young age that children often tease outsiders out of a sense of their own discomfort. Seldom do children understand the impact their taunts have on their victims. His parents avoided feeling inadequate and overwhelmed by ignoring the situation, reassuring themselves that Karl's isolation was just a temporary state of affairs. When children feel overwhelmed and frightened, they need adults to help them process their experiences in "bite-size pieces." Although his parents always cut Karl's meat for him, it never occurred to them he needed their help in a similar manner when it came to coping with painful emotions.

Karl excelled at athletics and, over time, was eventually accepted by his peers. His feelings of rejection were sealed over by the happiness and relief he experienced in his newfound friendships. When Kevin's ex-wife insulted Karl during that particularly vitriolic encounter, it set off an avalanche of buried feelings that Karl could only identify as a gripping anxiety he just couldn't shake.

As his resentment of Kevin began to take shape in his own mind, Karl became frightened by the possibility that he could explode in rage and drive Kevin away, just like ex-wife number two, as she was referred to by both men. As treatment progressed, Karl realized that Kevin's passivity, combined with the ex-wife's barbs, were seeds that fell on already fertile soil. The vulnerabilities he carried with him from childhood were exposed by this constellation of events and contributed to the disproportionately intense feelings of rejection he experienced. When Karl was ravaged by pain, both his earliest feelings of rejection and his resentment of Kevin were inaccessible to him. The pain effectively jammed his signals, and all he could experience was his pain. Although he was suffering physically, he was spared his unbearable feelings of worthlessness as well as the terrifying prospect of losing control of his anger.

Karl compared his anger to metastatic cancer, where one rogue cancer cell spreads uncontrollably throughout the body. Before long, the relentless course of the disease, like rage, decimates everything in its path. Therefore, to insure everyone's safety, Karl's body enforced the quarantine order against his anger, lest any destructive emotions escaped.

Unlike many other people with TMS, Karl did not ordinarily consider anger to be an indication of psychopathology, insanity, deviance, or a moral failing. In fact, he viewed anger as an inevitable part of life. Nonetheless he feared he could not regulate either his experiences or expressions of anger.

As he described it himself, he lacked internal speed bumps that could prevent him from accelerating from 0 to 60 in four seconds. Karl deemed it imperative for his own well-being to avoid ever "playing with matches." He had to renounce all anger like the alcoholic who completely and permanently abstains from alcohol to assure sobriety. Unfortunately, Karl confused sobriety with a dry drunk. A dry drunk is a state of sobriety enforced by white knuckling one's way to abstinence. The recovering alcoholic, on the other hand, comes to terms with the craving for alcohol, which compromises his self-control. So, Karl tried to obliterate any evidence of his own anger, rather than attempt to understand its menacing power to unravel him.

Karl appropriated a basic law of physics—two things cannot occupy the same space at the same time—in order to fireproof his psyche. His particularly severe TMS symptomatology precluded his attention to anything other than enduring his pain, monitoring the regimen of painkillers and radically circumscribing his activities in order not to provoke or exacerbate the pain.

Because Karl was oblivious to his own anger, he could innocently construe Kevin's distress as collateral damage to his own profound suffering, and not the result of his vengeful feelings. However, he was actually in less control over his anger because he had blinded himself to it. It turned out that ignorance wasn't bliss, and a lot more dangerous than playing with matches.

* * *

As part of Dr. Sarno's psychoeducational approach to treating TMS, he introduces patients to the Holmes and Rahe Scale (1998). The scale predicts a person's chances of developing a physical or emotional condition, based on cumulative exposure to stressful external events in the preceding year. Events range from mundane nuisances like getting a parking ticket to catastrophic events like the death of a spouse or the diagnosis of a life-threatening illness. The events are weighted: The parking ticket receives 1 point, the death of a spouse is assigned 50 points. Research indicates that when an individual accumulates more than 200 points in a year, he is at much greater risk of developing serious physical, emotional, or psychophysiologic conditions.

Although constitutional factors and personality variables play a role in an individual's vulnerability and resistance to stress, no one can imagine an individual entirely unscathed experiencing one or more of the following in the same year: the loss of a spouse, the amputation of a limb, an adult child's bitter divorce, or a hefty assessment by the co-op board.

Personality variables, childhood experiences, and external stressors all contribute to the development of TMS. The vignettes that follow focus on cases where external stressors are the most salient etiologic factor.

TMS as Adaptation to Stress

Rachel's daughter died a few weeks before her tenth birthday, after a five-year battle with leukemia. Rachel and her husband witnessed their daughter receive the Last Rites three times. Even though she was always anguished and exhausted, Rachel was never symptomatic with back pain. On the day of the funeral, Rachel developed acute back pain so disabling she could not stand to shower or dress herself without assistance. Her body was protesting and pleading, "I don't want to go to my daughter's funeral. I physically can't move. If I could move, then I could go to my daughter's funeral and would have to acknowledge she is dead and gone forever." Unfortunately, the etiology of Rachel's TMS was painfully apparent to everyone.

What was less apparent was the adaptive or survival value of Rachel's TMS symptomatology. If Rachel were to experience directly her agonizing loss, then she would have been flooded by feelings of traumatic intensity. If she drowned in her own sorrows, then the tragedy of her daughter's death would have been compounded by her inability to take care of her other children, who were also frightened and grief-stricken by the loss of their sister.

To avert an emotional blackout, Rachel developed severe TMS symptomatology. Although she was significantly debilitated physically, her cognitive functioning was preserved. So, in spite of her paralyzing grief, she could still oversee the care of her other children with support from others.

In Rachel's case, TMS also bought her time to master gradually the impact of her tragic loss. Mourning is a process that typically takes place over an extended period of time. The task of mourning is to reconcile eventually the experiences of letting go and holding on. If Rachel faced the enormity of her loss all at once, she would have been overrun by her grief. TMS symptomatology refocused her on literally putting one foot in front of the other. She was forced to concentrate on basic coping, so her emotional reserves could reconstitute themselves in preparation for mourning.

Obviously, if Rachel's TMS symptomatology persisted over an extended period, then its adaptive value would diminish. Instead of fostering the mourning process, at that point, it would be regarded as an impediment to resolving her feelings of loss. Fortunately, Rachel's back and leg pain subsided after several weeks. Like a brownout, her physical pain was a temporary emergency measure taken to ward off an even greater catastrophe without having to shut down her power grid completely.

* * *

Alex was plagued by recurrent sinus infections all throughout the winter and spring. The doctor recommended Alex get a CT scan to rule out the presence of a tumor, which might be interfering with the absorption of the antibiotics in his sinus cavities. Although the doctor emphasized that the likelihood of detecting such a tumor was extremely low, it wasn't non-existent, and Alex was appropriately panicked. Alex had been pain-free for several years following treatment for severe TMS involving his back and both legs. After completing the CT scan, the radiologist told him the results would not be available for several hours. He could wait for the results or get them from his doctor after the weekend.

Alex instinctively knew he could not tolerate waiting the weekend, since he felt his life could be in jeopardy. As soon as he decided to stay and wait it out, he envisioned plucking daisy petals to resolve the question, "She loves me, she loves me not." But the question he posed was, "Malignant or benign, malignant or benign?" As he pondered his future, he developed agonizing back pain for the first time in years. The pain was so severe it necessitated calling his wife, something he was reluctant to do lest he appear weak. After all, he was "merely waiting for test results." The pain distracted him from his anxiety, and his wife's presence comforted him. Also, the pain gave him no other choice but to wait for the results; he could hardly move. Alex finally received good news; there was no evidence of any kind of lesion. His TMS dissipated gradually over the next several days and Alex remained consistently asymptomatic with respect to his pain symptomatology.

* * *

Here again, TMS symptomatology rescues an individual from unbearable emotional distress. Always in the minds of individuals suffering from TMS, pain is the least horrible outcome amongst the alternatives available to them. However, for both Rachel and Alex, it is the preferred mode of dealing with emotional upheavals. It would be counterproductive for either Rachel or Alex to identify and reflect on their feelings at these crisis points, because their emotional experiences are actually nearly lethal in their intensity.

The majority of people with TMS genuinely fear the destructive powers of their emotional experiences. Often, these emotions are remnants of childhood fears, which have remained beyond the reach of their present day resources. If their adult experiences were integrated into these experiences, these feelings would not be nearly so threatening. For these individuals, TMS symptomatology protects them from deeply-felt, but nonetheless imaginary dangers, like the truly terrifying monsters lurking beneath children's beds.

External Stressors vs. Childhood Experience

On the day Isabel turned 65, she registered for Social Security benefits. On her trip home from registering, she developed back and leg pain, which she tried to ignore, attributing it to "getting older." The pain persisted despite her reliance on conservative treatments like bed rest, heating pads, and Motrin. She eventually consulted a physician, who ordered an MRI, which revealed arthritic changes in her lumbar spine. Nevertheless, she failed to respond to any of the recommended treatments, including a brief course of steroids, physical therapy, and finally two epidural injections. In desperation, she consulted Dr. Sarno, who informed Isabel that she was the poster girl for TMS.

At our first session, Isabel told me that she was strongly affected by Dr. Sarno's pithy observation, "aging is enraging." She told me how the day before her 65th birthday, she enjoyed visiting the art galleries in Soho and Chelsea. Now, just five weeks after that fateful day, she feels invisible when she makes her rounds of the latest shows. Obviously, she realized her perception was based on how she felt about herself and had nothing to do with how others regarded her. She asked, how could so much change, when in reality, nothing had changed except for the passage of five weeks? No one, she insisted, ages that much in five weeks! Her 65th birthday was the flash point for her diffuse, unformulated, and ever growing dread of aging.

To Isabel, and many others, aging means being relegated to the trash heap, being put out to pasture, all washed up, being told in effect, "You ain't what you used to be." When aging is officially acknowledged by registering for Social Security or being eligible for a half-fare transit pass, we are forced to confront our mortality. Many people become symptomatic with TMS when their own mortality is concretized by these rites of passage.

When Isabel was able to identify and express the feelings of anger, loss, and fear she experienced in relation to aging, she no longer was limited to expressing her distress solely through a body language of physical symptoms. This is not to say Isabel no longer feared her mortality or no longer yearned for her youth. Instead, she was now able to feel her feelings as feelings, as well as put them into words.

At the outset of treatment, Isabel regarded her feelings of rage over aging as childish and ungrateful. After all, no one is exempt from aging. She reasoned correctly that many regard the opportunity to age as a gift. As she came to realize that feelings are private, internal, emotional experiences and not inherently indicators of morality or character, she was better able to tolerate her negative feelings about aging without experiencing a loss of self-esteem.

* * *

Isabel's reaction to turning 65 highlights an important distinction between the effects of childhood experiences versus the etiological importance of external stressors. People often question, "Aren't the external stressors stressful because of your personality, which, after all, is an outgrowth of childhood experiences?" The simple, indeed overly simplistic answer is yes.

Childhood experiences are unique and specific. While many individuals have grown up in blended families, many others were reared in two-parent homes. Similarly, too many people have been the victims of bullying, but many others enjoyed immense popularity during their adolescent years. However, aging, loss, and physical jeopardy are external stressors of universal scope and reach. Certainly, how a particular individual reacts to these external stressors is largely determined by childhood experiences. If Rachel did not exhibit the typical TMS personality trait of taking care of others, she might have been more preoccupied with her own emotional depletion or the effect of her daughter's death on her marriage. No one would suggest that Rachel was unfazed by these other concerns. The hierarchy of her needs no doubt reveals the influences of her childhood. However, no one experiencing a tragic loss like Rachel's emerges unscathed. Devastation simply takes different forms. Anyone facing a potentially life-threatening diagnosis will be terrified. In fact, the absence of anxiety under such circumstances is a cause for alarm, not admiration. Again, the responses to terror are manifold: Some rearrange the deck chairs on the Titanic, others whistle a happy tune, and then there are those people who fortify themselves with drugs or alcohol, while others develop TMS.

There are many losses associated with aging. Isabel was especially attuned to her new status as a reluctantly invisible woman. Themes of being faceless in the crowd were painfully familiar to Isabel, growing up as the second oldest of eight children in a "catch as catch can" family. Aging provided a mirror to reflect these concerns; her early childhood experiences created them in the first place. Other people couldn't care less about invisibility because they are morbidly preoccupied with the loss of physical beauty and vitality, their own mortality, and the threat of increased dependency. Aging encompasses all of these potential losses, but childhood experiences sensitize the individual to particular ones.

American Academy of Pain Medicine, 12/26/2012, (http://www.painmed.org/patientcenter/facts_on_pain.aspx#refer).

Aron, L., & Anderson, F. S. (Eds.) (1998). *Relational Perspectives on the Body*. Hillsdale, NJ: The Analytic Press.

Deyo, R. (2004) *Breaking Down Back Pain*. Discovery Health TV.

Freud, S. (2005) *Studies on Hysteria*. New York: Basic Books.

Groopman, J. (2002). A Knife In The Back. *New Yorker*.

Groopman, J. (2007). *How Doctors Think*. Houghton Mifflin Company.

Masters, W., & Johnson, V. (1966). *Human Sexual Response*. New York: Bantam Books.

McDougall, J. (1989). *Theaters of the Body: A Psychoanalytic Approach to Psychosomatic Illness*. New York: W. W. Norton & Company.

Sarno, J. (1998). *The Mindbody Prescription*. Warner Books, Inc.

Sarno, J. (2006). *The Divided Mind*. Regan Books.

Schubiner, H. (2010). *Unlearn Your Pain*. Mind Body Publishing.

Sifneos, P. (1973). The Prevalence of "Alexithymic" Characteristics in Psychosomatic Patients. *Psychotherapy and Psychosomatics*.

van der Kolk, B. (1994). The Body Keeps The Score. *Harvard Review of Psychiatry*.

Frances Sommer Anderson

TREATING TMS PAIN: ILLUSTRATING THE CLINICAL PROCESS

Ranging from a treatment lasting 13 years to a focused consultation of five sessions over four days, I will describe both the intricacies of treating psychophysiologic symptoms as well as brief but substantive therapeutic interventions. Whenever possible, I use the patient's own words. Each of the six patients edited the chapters that you will read and approved the final manuscript. The chapters may be read in any order. For the reader's benefit, I will note that my work with Ellen and Mrs. R began in the early 1990s, after I had been working with Dr. Sarno's patients for11 years. The subsequent chapters present work dating from early 2000.

I begin by presenting excerpts from my first published work about treating TMS/PPD—Ellen's Story. The impact of the therapy was so memorable and evocative, I was compelled to write about it for a psychoanalytic text published in 1998. My collaboration with Ellen in the treatment and in writing offers lessons that I learn again and again in treating people with TMS/PPD pain and other somatic symptoms.

Mrs. R, who came for treatment after 40 years of pain symptoms, remained in therapy for 13 years, long after her presenting pain was relieved. The impact of our initial session was astounding for both of us. Subsequently, we discovered that overwhelming emotional experiences in early childhood, as well as in her 20s, had contributed to her long history of somatic complaints. Our work together was challenging and inspiring.

After Ellen and Mrs. R, I offer the outcome of a very brief, focused consultation with Kate, using a model that I have developed over many years for people who come to New York City from great distances and/or who have very tight time constraints. The power of this model will be evident as you read about our preparation for the consultation in my office and then the impact of the five sessions over four days. This consultation was followed by 8 Skype video consultations distributed over the next year.

Subsequently, I take the reader into the psychotherapy consulting room with Mr. L, Ms. T, and Mr. A. We follow their progress in recovering from physical symptoms by tracking the content of the sessions and their reports about their somatic states, often chronologically. I offer little or no discussion of the treatment process with these three patients, allowing the reader to be stimulated to question and reflect on the personal impact of this approach to treating TMS/PPD pain.

Becoming Aware of and Learning to Tolerate Overwhelming Emotions Relieves TMS Pain
Ellen's Story [4]

Ellen, now 46, was referred by Dr. Sarno, who told her that the musculoskeletal back pain she had experienced for nine years was due to Tension Myositis Syndrome, or TMS (later referred to as Tension Myoneural Syndrome by Dr. Sarno). During those nine years, Ellen had consulted numerous traditional and non-traditional health practitioners, always stopping short of surgery. None of the treatments had relieved her back pain. Her life had become quite constrained by the limits on physical activity that were prescribed by her physicians. In fact, she had developed fear of physical activity because she had come to believe that it would make her pain worse. In the interval between the TMS diagnosis and our initial consultation (about eight weeks), Ellen experienced a gradual and significant reduction in her pain level (she estimated a 35% reduction), and she began to resume physical activity. After the first three months of our work, she reported another pain reduction of about 40%, and she continued to increase her physical activities. The residual pain resolved by the end of the first year of treatment. Ellen and I identified a pattern of pain eruption during times of great emotional stress. The therapy process resolved the symptom within a few sessions, or sooner.

In the following discussion of my therapy with Ellen, I will demonstrate the process of resolving Tension Myositis

Syndrome across a period of several years of analytic work and within a single session, using dreams and other clinical material. I aim to illustrate (1) how feelings that could not be acknowledged and tolerated contributed to Ellen's physical symptoms; (2) how my awareness of my feelings in the therapy process, often at a somatic level, constituted a key element in the process of relieving the physical symptoms; and (3) by underscoring the challenge that patient and therapist face when their attempts to resolve physical symptoms result in serious, sometimes life-threatening illness. I will not discuss all of the psychodynamics because of the limited scope of this chapter.

I acknowledge, at the outset, Ellen's collaboration with me in the treatment process—through the journals that she kept during our work, through her active pursuit of knowledge of the mind-body relationship outside our sessions, and through her permission for me to use material from our endeavor in this chapter. I have included Ellen's own words whenever possible and integrated her editorial comments into the final text.

Feelings That Could Not Be Acknowledged and Tolerated: The Boxer Dog

The Tension Myositis diagnosis made sense to Ellen, so our analytic work began—eight years before I wrote this chapter in 1996. At that time, Ellen had been divorced from her husband, Ted, for nine years. Her parents were living and she has one sibling, a brother, Joe, who is three years older. She was living alone and had had a married lover, Mark, for nine years.

The therapy process started for me as I listened to Ellen's voice on her answering machine when I returned her initial call. Her way of speaking had an immediate impact: Her voice was flat, her pace was slow, deliberate, and measured. As we spoke in the initial interview, I noticed that she paused frequently and swallowed audibly. After a few sessions, I realized that her speech pattern was heightening my awareness of her lack of emotional response to what I was often experiencing as highly emotionally-charged material. I often felt tense at these times, recognizing stirrings of anger or outrage or disappointment that I, the therapist, could not express as Ellen described various interpersonal situations that had turned out badly for her.

Early in the treatment I began to feel mildly distressed that Ellen was not experiencing feelings that she needed to feel in order to take care of her needs and protect herself in interactions with people. For example, I noticed that she spoke in great detail about her relationship with her ex-husband, Ted, with almost no emotional response as she talked about the way their marriage had failed and about the numerous ways that she continued to be involved in his life, even after he had remarried and had two children. I remember being especially surprised to hear that she had used her considerable talent as a landscape architect to specify the plantings for the grounds of Ted's new family's home, only a few houses away from her own. Given how painful she said that their break-up had been, I wondered silently how she could continue to be involved in his new marriage in such an intimate way, especially since her own intimate life with a partner had continued to be frustrating and largely unfulfilling. How could she tolerate these interactions? Weren't they at least somewhat painful? Ellen also described work and other personal situations in which she appeared not to be experiencing a sense that her own interests could be endangered by the agendas of colleagues and friends. Meanwhile, quite early, I was already able to anticipate that Ellen was going to get "hurt" in interpersonal relationships because she was apparently unable to use knowledge of past experience that could help her protect herself.

I was familiar with this apparent "absence of feelings," having encountered it frequently during the previous 18 years treating people who have TMS pain. When working with a patient referred with a diagnosis of Tension Myositis Syndrome, reaching the "emotions" or "feelings" is usually a fundamental part of the analytic process. With Ellen, I guessed that a big challenge lay ahead because her "absence of feelings" was so striking and because my somatic response to her was so strong: While I waited eagerly, yet apprehensively, to hear what was to happen next, I would often feel a visceral sense of dread and notice an increase in my heart rate. At the same time, I would often be holding my breath, which I have learned is my unconscious somatic response when I do not want to fully experience my emotional reactions.

A dream that Ellen brought after five months of treatment will illustrate further this aspect of her psychological functioning, my response to it, and the implications for making sense of her musculoskeletal pain. First, I will summarize the context in therapy in which she brought the dream. We had been identifying the emotional circumstances in which her back pain had started and persisted. Briefly, Ellen's back pain had begun about six months after her divorce from Ted was final—after a separation of about a year and a half. She had described that separation as a period of unrelenting activity that therapists recognize as a way of protecting oneself from feelings. In her words, "I was a human doing, not a human being." We had come to understand that this activity had been, unconsciously, a way to avoid dealing with her emotional reactions to the marital separation and the pending loss of the marriage.

I had also learned that, through her marriage to Ted after college at age 22, she had gained a place of respect in her family for the first time. She had remarked several times that she felt that her mother was "in love" with Ted and that he had found in her mother the kind of maternal care and attention that was not available to him from his own mother. Ellen had also reported that the only support her family gave her was to take the "wife/mommy track," despite her obvious considerable talent in two professional areas. In our initial session, in fact, she had stated that her family had always "championed" (her word) her brother, Joe. She felt that they had never championed her.

While Ellen was married to Ted, she worked full-time to support him through his post-graduate professional training and went to school at night for a Master's degree in one area of interest. Ted was actively discouraging and disparaging of her efforts to get this degree; her parents were ambivalent. When Ted completed his degree, she could not overcome his active discouragement of her pursuing additional career goals and settled for work in a variety of situations in which she always felt frustrated and unfulfilled. When she separated from Ted, at his request and to her family's dismay, she felt, in her words, "like throwing myself on the railroad tracks" because of the shame and the enormous threat to her self-image. Ted's stated reasons for wanting a divorce was that Ellen was too "controlling" of him in her need for "neatness" and "cleanliness" in their household. As the divorce was approaching, and prior to the onset of her back pain, Ellen had been preparing to enter a training program to get a long-cherished professional credential. She had to relinquish this goal after the onset of the debilitating back pain and a subsequent fracture to her left arm when she was hit by a motorcyclist. Forced to find a new career path, she entered a profession that is still chosen predominantly by men.

Ellen told the following dream at the beginning of a session, introducing it by saying that she'd had a "nightmare":

I was out in the countryside somewhere, riding bikes with Ted. It started out pleasant. We had a boxer dog with us. My family got one, a male, when I was six months old and we had it till I was seven. The second boxer was when I was in fourth grade and we had it till I was a junior in high school—a female. Both became overprotective and we had to get rid of them. Ted and I were in Minnesota for three years and then we came to Princeton and after one year we bought a house. The neighbors had two boxers. The fawn one lived with us in the evenings. Shortly before we broke up, one morning we found him dead on our porch—rat poison. The dog in the dream was nice-looking—running along with us. The first part was euphoric. Somewhere in the middle, the dog was not keeping up. I knew it was sick. It keeled over dead, rolled over on its back, its chest cavity was open and deteriorated.

As I listened, the tension mounted for me but Ellen

seemed very calm. She had told me that this was a nightmare. I was wondering, "What's going to happen?" The way she was interweaving the history of the boxers was heightening the tension by delaying the nightmare ending. I also noticed that there was no detectable change in her emotional state as she told this "nightmare." There was just Ellen, in her calm, measured tones, telling me the story.

When she finished telling this dream, she continued by giving more useful factual associations, in her now familiar detached, objective manner. Meanwhile, the image of the damaged, dead boxer persisted for me as I cringed inside and wanted to clutch my chest protectively. I was wondering what had happened to the boxer, what could this signify? What had happened in the marriage that I hadn't heard about? Why was euphoria followed by—by what? Followed by physical trauma to the boxer dog and what I experienced as a blank space where I had expected to hear an emotional response. Meanwhile, I silently filled in the gap—I was horrified. Nothing in our discussions to date, nothing in the "facts" she had provided, had given me any indication that her experience in the marriage had been this traumatic.

As I listened to her associations to the dream, I waited for her to show some feeling for the boxer, clearly an important attachment figure given her story, but she showed none. Also, I still wasn't clear what had made it a nightmare for her. Finally, I wondered aloud what her reaction was to what had happened to the boxer. She looked stunned, she was speechless, and she couldn't find a reaction to report.

This was an early pivotal moment in the treatment, one to which we referred often. One of my roles as therapist was taking shape—I was to register emotional responses when Ellen showed none, or none that I deemed appropriate, that is. Through my silent, but visceral, feeling response to hearing about the physical trauma to the boxer, I was entering a lengthy process with Ellen: I would silently experience pain and rage for the boxer and Ellen, as she represented herself again and again as a sick and damaged boxer in her dreams, and as she described herself over and over as the victim of aggression in interpersonal relationships. Early in the treatment, she would report this information to me with apparently little reaction, while I was left holding all the violent images and their associated emotions and trying to find a way to make sense of the origins of such violent, physically destructive aggression.

I want to refer to what happened in this session as an example of extreme disconnection of "cognitive awareness" from "emotional experiencing." Specifically—in this dream, Ellen had "cognitive awareness" that something was wrong with the boxer. The dream ended as she was "observing" what was wrong, but she showed no emotional response to that knowledge. One of my early roles as Ellen's therapist was to register and tolerate painful and violent feelings that she had been unable to detect and tolerate.

When Ellen told this dream, and I heard what had happened to the boxer and noted her lack of emotional response, I immediately speculated that there was a significant relationship between her persistent back pain and what had happened to the boxer. I conjectured that she was portraying in the image of the damaged, dead boxer dog some kind of traumatic experience of which neither she nor I was yet aware. I hypothesized that the blank space that I experienced in Ellen's telling of the dream referred to her failure to be aware of an emotional response to what had happened with Ted. I wondered if her inability to fully acknowledge what had happened in the marriage and her inability to mourn the loss of Ted had led to back pain; in other words, I wondered if the back pain had come to serve as a powerful protection from intolerable feelings.

It was not until one and a half years later that Ellen began to fill in that "gap," when she began to disclose, very slowly, traumatic experiences with Ted that she "knew" about but had not been able to "feel." In a session near the 11th anniversary of her divorce, she mentioned fleetingly that he had been physically violent toward her. Disclosing this fact, without any details, was retraumatizing: Not only did she have to relive the experience in reporting it, but she also felt tremendous shame and humiliation that the violence had occurred. Perhaps worse, she felt that she was betraying Ted.

Months later, I learned that Ted had once hit her in the chest in a violent outburst: We had finally made a link between the decayed chest of the dream boxer and a violent physical and emotional experience that happened in the marriage. Still later, she revealed that she was, in her words, "living in danger the whole time." To keep him from "flying off the handle," she felt like she was "stretching a rubber band as far as possible." "Just to sleep with somebody with that kind of violence is unreal," she said. When I asked how she was able to do it, she replied, "I kept myself in a bloody straitjacket."

In June, 1994, the O. J. Simpson story triggered an apparent reliving of the violence with Ted, when Ellen developed a sudden, intense relationship with a man she met in a singles bar. He quickly became emotionally violent and controlling, and there was reason to believe that he could be physically violent as well. In this stressful emotional context, Ellen developed a serious abdominal infection of unknown etiology, her second such condition during the analysis. This infection required hospitalization and prevented her from having intercourse with this man. In our analysis of this repetition and my overprotective reactions during it, we elaborated further the violence that she experienced with her ex-husband. Ellen stated, "When Ted took my life in his hands, I had no reaction. The mindset I had was that it didn't matter. When he hit me, I thought I dreamed it." The power of disconnecting from feelings in order to survive can hardly be more evocatively described. These vivid images helped us make even more sense of her chronic pain and its relationship to the underlying fear and rage that she could not experience.

The immediate frightening physical consequences of experiencing overwhelming emotions associated with traumatic material in sessions has underscored for me the importance of working very slowly and carefully to help Ellen learn to tolerate threatening emotions that are activated during the therapy process. Ellen strongly agreed that I needed to underscore caution in this discussion. Analysts have always been advised to proceed carefully when treating somatic symptoms (e.g., Krystal, 1988; McDougall, 1985, 1989). I have been made acutely aware that the impact of the therapy process is paradoxical in that our very attempts to treat the condition underlying symptoms can also prove painful and sometimes perilous.

Learning to Recognize and Tolerate Feelings: The Rabbits

To further illustrate our psychological understanding of Ellen's physical symptoms, I will discuss a dream that she brought about one year after the preceding dream. She told it at the end of a session where the theme had been "keeping secrets." She introduced the dream by talking about a movie—*The Prince of Tides*—that she had seen the night that she had the dream. Her remarks focused on the "enduring relationship" that the central male character had with the female psychiatrist/analyst. She had cried for hours after seeing the movie. She also noted that she had had an intense conflictual phone interaction with her brother the day before the session. Then she said, "My back started to hurt when I started to tell you the dream."

> I was in Switzerland, skiing, which I don't do now. I learned to ski with Ted the first year we were married. We were skiing, trying to get on one lift to go to a scenic run. We missed it, got on another one. We were skiing through mountains, we paused. I looked over and I could see a tiny white rabbit. A rabbit sitting inside the carcass of a twin bunny. It was dead. The first rabbit was eating the carcass of the rabbit it was sitting in. It pushed the dead rabbit off the cliff. A bloody scene. The live rabbit was sitting on the edge of the cliff wriggling its nose. A harmless, cute rabbit that had done this deed. Ted and I were watching. Three or four ugly men came up and confronted us. It's giving me a chill to tell you. The dream shifted. I

was with my family—mother, father, brother, my family of origin. We were watching a home movie documentary about the white rabbit eating the carcass. When it ended, I was sitting on the floor. I had a leather-embossed story book with the words "My Story" on the cover. I had a Windex bottle in the shape of a little girl. I was spraying it clean, only the cover.

There, my back doesn't hurt so much.

First, I want to note Ellen's progress in processing troubling experiences. Specifically, in this dream, Ellen moves from being merely an onlooker at a scene of disturbing physical violence, to portraying herself as the subject of the violence: She takes the scene of trauma to the rabbit's body into her family home where it becomes "Her Story." But, as in many previous boxer dreams, she is still telling "Her Story" with animals as the characters representing the trauma.

Although Ellen reports no emotional reaction within the dream, this time she tells me that her back started to hurt when she started to tell me the dream. This time, she knows there's a connection between her body's reaction and the content and telling of the dream. She's learned to read her body's signals, an important first step on the road to eliminating the physical symptoms. Further, she gets a "chill" while telling the dream—this time, I was not alone in feeling a visceral response to the horror of the dream image. Then, Ellen says she feels better after telling me the dream—another linking of mind and body.

In the five and a half years of therapy since this dream, Ellen and I have continued to understand the significance one of her "secrets" —the theme of violence in her family, the violence she depicts in the many damaged boxer dream images and in the image of the horror and destruction of the rabbit that becomes "Her Story." To date, the clinical material has pointed us to Ellen's powerful, conflictual attachment to her brother, Joe, three years older.

Ellen seems to have received highly contradictory messages from her parents about her status in the family compared with Joe's, reflected, for example, in many dreams about "unequal playing fields." Her increasing awareness of this has been an extremely painful theme running throughout our work. She recalls, from an early age, family stories about her mother's first pregnancy that ended in the miscarriage of a male child. Further, she has been told that both parents were hoping that she would be a boy and that they had chosen a name for him in their eager anticipation of his birth.

She has always felt that Joe is the favored sibling, whom she also adored, whose cowboy outfits she wore when he outgrew them, and whose toys she preferred to hers. One source of confusion was that her parents did not make an appropriate age and "sexual" differentiation between her and Joe—in many ways, they treated them as "twin boys." On the other hand, she felt that her mother treated Joe preferentially, exemplified in a letter that she had written to Joe when she was in first grade. It read: "I love you but you be bad to me. Mom gets me and lets you free." When Ellen read my manuscript, she told me that my including this letter was the most painful disclosure for her, but she felt strongly that I must include it because it was such a critical piece of information about "Her Story."

It was not until much later in the treatment that we began to appreciate just how painful the relationship with Joe had been. I have learned about scenes of emotional and physical conflict with Joe that Ellen has depicted in the following way: "My parents would let stuff go on till I screamed in pain and would get hurt." "I knew I was going to get picked on, I just never knew when. My whole life with my brother was that way. They were right there letting it happen, so the violation was more intense." She would rail out to her parents, "How can you let him do this?" but they would not intervene.

In writing this chapter, I became aware that I was not adequately clear what the "stuff" was that went on with Joe. I had not been able to pursue it further because of time constraints on our therapy that Ellen and I were experiencing due to her dire financial circumstances. When Ellen and I discussed my lack of knowledge in this area, she identified two kinds of "stuff" that went on: sibling competition regarding physical strength (e.g., "You can't bend my finger back") and verbal combat (e.g., Joe would tease her by calling her a "stupid" girl and refer to her as "my idiot sister" when she took too long in the family's only bathroom).

When Ellen gave me these examples in the session, I could see that she was starting to be overwhelmed with emotional pain, as her eyes filled with tears and her neck and face reddened, and I remembered that sessions like this would often be followed by a severe somatic reaction—usually an infection. Here I was reminded of Laub and Auerhahn's (1993) description of the dilemma we all face in dealing with trauma. They state: "We all hover at different distances between knowing and not knowing about trauma, caught between the compulsion to complete the process of knowing and the inability or fear of doing so" (p. 288). Further, they point out: "To protect ourselves from [feelings] we must, at times, avoid knowledge" (p. 288). Our interaction in this session acutely exemplifies this dilemma. As the session progressed, Ellen acknowledged that she was feeling overwhelmed, and said that she thought we should go more slowly. I agreed. In the discussion that followed, she asked me if I thought that I had been afraid to know more about some areas of her experience. I answered that I thought that was likely, given the number of instances when I had failed to ask for details about her early conflictual encounters with Joe, for example.

Because the information that Ellen and I had at the writing of this chapter still does not adequately account for the degree of violence and bodily damage in her dream images and in her physical illnesses, I have to question what more there is to learn. Nevertheless, Ellen's gradual ownership of the traumatic experience with Joe that we do "know" about has increased her awareness of how she leaves herself open to boundary violations in the present. She has begun to realize, with great shame and fear, that she has repeated these scenarios with Joe in her relationship with Ted, with her married lover, and in other personal and professional relationships.

In the therapy, we have learned that for Ellen, experiencing anger/rage can be emotionally overwhelming and somatically dangerous. In a session where she tried to recall whether she'd ever felt angry at her brother, she said, "My mind just went." She "saw red," and almost blacked out, stating that anger at Joe "looms as a convulsion."

Ellen's fear of interpersonal confrontation was also vividly illustrated to us in a dream in which she was riding with her family in the family car. She was angry about what was happening in the car and decided to get out and walk. When she got out, she asked her mother to get her suitcase from the car trunk. When her mother handed her the suitcase, Ellen threw it at her. When Ellen told this dream in the session, she almost "blacked out" when she started to experience the rage that she felt toward her mother. We learned that she was fearful that she would destroy her mother and was ashamed that she experienced such destructive impulses toward her mother. These "aggressive" and "destructive" versions of her "self" were overwhelming. She stated, "This is why I get back pain and get sick, because I don't use this realm." "I'm afraid to use (healthy) boxer emotions, afraid to make the connection." At these junctures, Ellen has frequently reported that she "can't think and feel at the same time."

When Ellen refers to "healthy boxer emotions" in this context, she is referring to the optimum use of anger and aggression in interpersonal relationships, as well as anger at me when I confront her if I sense that she is not taking care of herself in interpersonal situations. After five years of therapy, she said, "You're less of an authority figure now. This is a revolution. Previously I was looking for mirroring, now I'm looking for arguing." However, she was still frightened of losing closeness with me, afraid of destroying a positive connection with me if she experiences and expresses anger at me, as she did with her mother in the preceding dream. In exploring her experience of feeling angry at me, she has said, "You're the first person for the longest period who supported me." "If I showed anger at you...we'd be equal combatants on the playing field. Instead, I become a stone. The only time I can remember summoning anger at you, I got a little terse tone. I squeezed shut the floodgate, contracted the gluteus maximus. I don't let my anger out and screw up my back instead. I can't reverse it all at once." We continued to identify and analyze Ellen's anger and aggression toward me. This is always an aspect of the psychodynamic psychotherapy process, but it is particularly important for a severely somatizing person like Ellen, for whom rage and aggression could not be experienced directly for a considerable period, resulting in severe body symptoms.

The Therapist's Emotional Participation as a Crucial Element in Symptom Resolution

In our relationship, it was essential for me to tolerate hearing about situations that evoked painful, frightening, violent feelings, the first step in helping Ellen tolerate experiencing these emotions. If our pace was too quick, she became ill, much like the boxers in her dreams. In describing our roles in the early phase of the analysis, Ellen said, "I'll tell you in monotone, with no inflection in my voice. I can pass it through you. Once I pass it through you, the jig is up. I have to feel it." Thus, the boxers also represented feelings that she needed to experience. I, in the role of the boxer, have had to suffer a great deal as we explored such violent, bodily destructive dream images as the boxer who vomited a half-decayed capon and had a bowel movement of two whole, half-decayed turkey carcasses containing three half-decayed rats; the boxer who was knocked senseless in a violent fight with another dog; and the boxer who was injured by a stake in her back and went into convulsions and died because of the pain.

To explain further the importance of my emotional response to Ellen, I include, on her recommendation, a boxer dream from an early phase of our work, which has always been in the background but never adequately understood. The dream occurred shortly after Ellen's hospitalization (the first during the treatment) for a life-threatening pelvic infection, initially thought to be toxic shock syndrome but later stated to be "of unknown etiology." This infection occurred about three weeks after her mother's hysterectomy for uterine cancer.

In the week prior to the onset of the acute infection, we had a session in which Ellen experienced the realization intensely, for the first time, that the very bedrock of her identity had been to bear the emotional pain for others, in particular her mother, her ex-husband, and her married lover, Mark. She almost fainted on the couch just before she articulated her situation in this way: "I abandoned my body and soul and jumped into theirs." While she was in the hospital, we arranged for a phone session on a weekend day, and she called me at my home office. In that session, she revealed that she had felt suicidal after she left the session where she had had the painful insight about a primary source of her self-esteem. Soon after the phone session, she had a dream in which she came to visit me in my home in New York City (she lives outside the city). She opened the door to my home and let my four boxers run out into the street.

After reading my disclosures about the emotional pain I have experienced during the analysis, Ellen said that she finally understood the dream about my boxers. She conjectured that, early on, she must have been aware that I was reacting to "Her Story" and that she must have unconsciously needed me to feel for her in order that she could begin to tolerate feeling it herself. Certainly, my concern for her was apparent during the somatic aftermath of the traumatic session.

The importance of my showing feelings became clearer to both of us when we discussed Ellen's reaction to reading my description of her voice as "flat." At first, she was surprised and hurt. On further reflection, she realized that this aspect of her speech pattern has probably been interpreted by friends and others as an indication that she is very "laid back" and able to tolerate a great deal of upset. She also appreciated, for the first time, that neither of her parents show a range of emotional reactions. Only her brother, Joe, recognizably expresses feelings, particularly anger, as did her ex-husband, Ted. She speculated that her parents' narrow range of emotional expression had impaired the development of her own emotional functioning, leaving her unprepared to recognize and tolerate feelings, particularly anger.

Summary

Ellen came for treatment because of bodily pain that was persistent and disabling. From my therapist's perspective, this kind of bodily experience presents a compelling challenge and sometimes frightening dangers. In the preceding discussion, I have shown that Ellen was extremely disconnected from the emotional significance of a great deal of her life experiences. I illustrated our discovery in the therapy process that this disconnection had resulted in somatic symptoms—musculoskeletal pain and a variety of infections of varying degrees of severity.

In this chapter, I also documented how somatic symptoms appear and can be resolved in the treatment process. In the first few months of the therapy, Ellen's musculoskeletal pain essentially resolved, and she resumed most of the physical activities that she had previously avoided on the instruction of her physicians. I also reported that she occasionally experienced a return of the back pain when greatly stressed (e.g., her back pain returned as she prepared to tell me the "rabbit" dream, and the pain remitted as she finished telling me the dream). Further, I noted with caution that in the process of understanding the meanings of the symbol of the boxer dog, twin rabbits, and other dream images, new and frightening symptoms, usually infections, appeared. I consider this an indication that the treatment process is extremely powerful and that it must continue, even more carefully and cautiously.

The psychotherapeutic quest that Ellen and I undertook strikingly demonstrates the power of our emotions to affect our physical health. Ellen reported that her debilitating musculoskeletal back pain of nine years was reduced by 35% two months after she received a medical diagnosis that linked her emotional life with her physical symptoms. After three months of psychoanalytic treatment, she reported another pain reduction of about 40%. As the analysis unfolded, Ellen developed sudden, severe infections of unknown etiology following sessions in which traumatic emotions were experienced. This kind of power can be "empowering" to therapist and patient, and it can be frightening. Again, I caution slow and careful therapeutic work when a patient enters treatment with a long history of somatic symptoms.

In our journey, Ellen and I discovered the importance of the therapist's ability to tolerate painful and violent emotions. I believe that this aspect of the treatment process has been overlooked, especially in the treatment of people with musculoskeletal back pain. The analyst is challenged to consider, "How much pain can I, and am I willing, to tolerate as my analytic partner learns, or seems not to learn, through his/her experience what is painful and how much s/he can and should tolerate?" I learned that Ellen felt that I still am not always able to "stay with her" as she describes more situations in which she is treated with disrespect and hostility. She recently said that all she wants from me is to tolerate being with her in the moment when she is struggling to make a decision about a course of action to take. We have identified that sometimes I am the one who disconnects, for example, by registering discomfort directly, through a change in the tone of my voice, and/or by interpreting her "self-destructive tendencies" prematurely.

Ellen reminded me of a dream in which she was rushing to get on a commuter train and saw that I was already on the train. The door closed as she rushed to enter. She readily interpreted the dream in terms of our therapy relationship: "You get on the train without me." I have been challenged to look inward to understand my resistance to "staying with her" as she discovers disconnected longing and anger/rage. I have had to confront my family's history of grief and rage and the ways it has contributed to my own tendencies to disconnect, as well as the ways in which it has enabled me to be attuned to the emotional functioning of my patients.

The exacting process of understanding the psychological underpinnings of physical symptoms often proved viscerally, emotionally, painful for me and sometimes perilous for Ellen. In her words, "It'll make you crazy to feel 40 years of what was repressed in such a concentrated fashion. I'm afraid I'll go mad [like one of the dream boxers] if I feel the pain." Nevertheless, Ellen's courage and determination were inspiring. She stated, "When I come to the session, I bring a bag of courage. Let's go." It seems to me that our therapy process was, in large part, a kind of "championing" of Ellen by attempting to tolerate hearing about "Her Story," to stay in the room with her as she is trying to tell us. In giving me permission to share our work in this chapter, Ellen said that she hopes that her experience, presented in this way, will prove helpful to others. Our shared belief in the benefits of attempting to recognize and tolerate feelings in order to relieve physical symptoms has helped us endure and prevail.

---

[4] This section includes excerpts from the chapter, "Psychic Elaboration of Musculoskeletal Back Pain: Ellen's Story," published in *Relational Perspectives on the Body: Psychoanalytic Theory and Practice*, edited by Lewis Aron & Frances Sommer Anderson (The Analytic Press, 1998). Permission was granted by Taylor & Francis Group, LLC to update and revise the excerpts that were published in that psychoanalytic text.

Overwhelming Experiences in Childhood and Adulthood

Sessions with Mrs. R

Mrs. R and I worked together over a period of 13 years, on a once- to twice-a-week schedule. We explored the relationship between musculoskeletal pain and feelings that had been difficult, sometimes impossible, for her to experience before coming for therapy. Indeed, at the beginning, she was often unable to detect what she felt when discussing issues that seemed to me to be highly emotional. In what follows, I will be illustrating how Mrs. R's pain was relieved when she was able to experience her feelings about what she was discussing.

Mrs. R came to see me at age 61 because of recurrent musculoskeletal foot, shoulder, hip, and back pain that she had since her early 20s. During that 40-year history of pain, she had consulted many medical specialists, who had prescribed numerous interventions. She had tried many of them but had found no permanent relief.

Let me introduce you to Mrs. R and to the therapy process by telling you about the first two sessions.

In the initial consultation, I asked Mrs. R to describe the physical symptoms that brought her to see me, and I asked questions that would define the "emotional" context in which she began to experience pain. For example, I asked how old she was, where she lived, and with whom, along with other questions that would help us identify what stresses she was experiencing at that time. You will see from the description that follows how we begin to assess the level of stress and her emotional response to it. We are trying to find connections between her emotional life and the development of her physical symptoms.

Mrs. R reported that she had had foot pain since her second oldest daughter's wedding, six months ago. She had also developed stabbing, gnawing pain in her right shoulder. She had had similar physical symptoms since her early 20s. I asked what was happening at that time, around 40 years ago. She was newly married to a husband who worked very long hours as a young professional, leaving her alone with no friends in an unfamiliar city. She mentioned the stress of adjusting to the demands of motherhood, noting that she has four children, three girls and a boy. I asked their ages.

After a long pause, she said, "You know, I had another child," and started to weep. "My first child, a boy, had spina bifida.[5] He lived 12 years. I never saw him." I could feel that she was distressed that she was weeping in the presence of a stranger: She remarked several times, through her tears, that she could not believe that she had told me about her son, that she had had no thought of him before the interview, and that she did not understand why she was crying.

When she regained enough composure to continue the interview, she told me that she had mononucleosis during the pregnancy and was sure that was the cause of the spina bifida. Then she surprised me by saying, "Maybe this explains why I've been so attentive to my other children," and elaborated briefly about how attentive and engaged she has been with each child. As her tears subsided, she told me more about her family of origin. She has a brother four years older, whom she referred to as a "genius." She described her sister, six years younger, as a "little limited in her abilities."

As we approached the end of the interview, Mrs. R started to weep again and told me that she had developed severe migraines and foot pain the year after her first son was born. Her husband and the doctors had decided that she should not see him, and they had placed him in a residential setting without consulting her. As the session ended, she remarked again, with astonishment, that she could not believe that she had told me about her son and that she did not understand why she became so upset.

Deeply moved by her story, I was wondering what Mrs. R had endured all these years regarding her first-born. I was also concerned that her spontaneous disclosure to a stranger, accompanied by unanticipated intense feelings, would generate so much emotional discomfort that she wouldn't return, even though she had made an appointment for a second session. In many sessions that followed, I wondered how much emotional pain I was causing Mrs. R, and I worried that the feelings that came up during our explorations might become so difficult to tolerate that she would leave. To paraphrase what many of my patients who have TMS have said, "I'd rather have my TMS than tolerate this emotional pain!" I want to emphasize here that no matter how motivated you may be to overcome TMS, you may falter when you begin to acknowledge and experience feelings that you have sequestered in your emotional reservoir for many, many years. In Mrs. R's case, for 40 years.

Mrs. R arrived for our second session, elated, saying that she could not remember when she had felt better physically. As a matter of fact, she had played tennis for the first time in many months. Silently, I, too, was elated. I was also surprised at her resilience—and encouraged by it. As I would usually do, I asked what she thought had made her feel better. She said it had something to do with talking about her first son, but she did not know exactly how it was related.

I took this opportunity to ask more questions about what had happened after he was born. She disclosed that she had been "depressed" for several months, but she and her husband never spoke about him. As soon as possible, they had another child, and she experienced considerable apprehension during that second and the succeeding three pregnancies. Her husband visited their son regularly, but she could not remember how often. They never discussed his visits. The only details she wanted to know were the color of his hair—red—and his name—Steven. She had somehow learned that he had an enlarged head, due to the hydrocephaly often associated with spina bifida, and that he was confined to a wheelchair. She did not want to know more and tried hard not to let herself picture him in any more detail. She had never spoken with her other children about him, and was not sure if her husband had told them that they had another sibling.

I was tense throughout the session, feeling that I had to constrain my inquiry about Steven and her reactions to losing him because she had been so distressed in our first meeting. I did not want to push her too far, but I also needed to pursue her. Like many of my patients with TMS who like to feel "in control" of their emotions, it was clear that she preferred a composed demeanor: She shed no tears in the second session. Despite her palpable reserve, however, I could feel that she was determined to participate in the therapy process. Her relief from years of bodily pain after the first session had apparently convinced her that this approach could be helpful. I silently admired her courage and tenacity.

In the second session, I also inquired about her sister's "somewhat limited abilities." She offered that Alexa was slightly retarded, probably because of an accident at age two, when Mrs. R was around eight years old. The accident was at the family's country house in the summer. Mrs. R was watching over her sister in an upstairs bedroom. Even though there must have been a nanny present, Alexa fell out of the window. Mrs. R stated, "I was never blamed for it, but the family always said that Alexa was never the same after the concussion." Before her parents died, she promised them that she would always take care of Alexa. We had now identified a second, longstanding source of Mrs. R's unconscious rage—taking care of Alexa. She described her as extremely self-centered and insensitive to others' feelings and needs, in stark contrast to Mrs. R's empathic nature.

We spent considerable time in therapy discussing her relationship with Alexa. To summarize, we linked some of her musculoskeletal pains to hateful, angry, often rageful feelings toward Alexa that she had been unable to experience prior to her work with me. Because these feelings did not fit with Mrs. R's image of herself as patient, compassionate, and willing to fulfill her promise to her parents, they were banished to her emotional reservoir. Recognizing these feelings and learning to tolerate them resulted in considerable relief of her pain.

As Mrs. R became able to tolerate feeling angry at Alexa, we discussed the possibility that she could re-evaluate the level of care that she was giving Alexa. She was able to consider setting some limits on Alexa's self-centered, presumptuous demands on Mrs. R's time, as well as Alexa's intrusions into Mrs. R's personal and family space. We discussed the concept of "boundaries," both emotional and physical. For example, Alexa felt free to show up at her sister's home in the city and in the country at any time, unannounced, apparently oblivious to the household's routines. She often parked her car in Mrs. R's driveway, seemingly unaware that she was blocking her sister's family members' exit. Mrs. R felt she couldn't speak up to Alexa in either of these situations. As you read these examples and imagine yourself in Mrs. R's shoes, what would you feel, and what would you do about what you feel? Could you allow yourself to feel furious at Alexa? Would you feel guilty having the thought of setting limits for her?

Check in with yourself about your emotional reactions to what you've learned thus far. What would you say about the lingering aftershocks of Mrs. R's traumatic experience with Alexa in childhood? Might she have felt responsible for the accident even though she was not blamed for it? Could rage about carrying such a heavy load of responsibility since childhood have contributed to Mrs. R's TMS? Now, consider this experience in childhood together with the traumatic loss of Mrs. R's first-born child. What do you imagine that you would feel? Can you estimate the intensity of shame, guilt, and rage that you might feel—a potent combination of feelings, often repressed because of that very potency?

In the remainder of this chapter, I will focus on the issue of Mrs. R's first-born child to show how challenging it can be for someone to feel threatening feelings and how not feeling them can result in TMS symptoms.

As the psychotherapy process continued, on a once- to twice-weekly basis, I had many thoughts about Steven. I had treated children and adults with spina bifida when I worked in physical rehabilitation medicine at Rusk Institute. I could not help picturing him in a wheelchair, with red hair and hydrocephaly. I wondered what his body looked like at each developmental stage. How mobile was he? Was he incontinent of bowel and bladder? How had his intelligence been affected by the hydrocephaly? How did he die? The therapist's curiosity is an important element in the treatment process because the patient may not be able to be conscious of their own curiosity. We're all familiar with the expression, "I can't bear to think about it," used when the feelings associated with the thoughts about a subject would be too difficult to bear. We can understand that it had been too painful for Mrs. R to "think" about Steven very often. In this situation, the therapist has to "think the unthinkable" and carefully check to see if the patient has ever had such thoughts.

In sessions with Mrs. R, I often hesitated to bring up the subject of Steven, wondering if I was making too much of the loss of her son. I was also reluctant to cause her emotional pain by asking about him. I watched her dreams for signs of him and found fragments: The arm of a wheelchair; something red dripping down from the attic of the country house where a mother squirrel had abandoned her babies; a very large head floating in space. Even though, to me, these images seemed associated with details she "knew" about Steven, when I was alone in a session with Mrs. R, I could easily lose my conviction that they were relevant. Aside from asking her what came to her mind when she focused on each image, I rarely commented on my thoughts about these dream elements. I waited until I felt she was able to tolerate feelings that might arise if she consciously associated these images with Steven.

Now, I will take you with me into a session with Mrs. R, eight years after treatment began. I want to demonstrate how we established that sealing off emotions, particularly about Steven, led to her TMS pain. As she experienced her feelings, she began to experience relief from her physical symptoms.

It is January 9. Mrs. R, trim and athletic, enters briskly and gives a big sigh as she settles into a chair facing me. She has a repertoire of sighs and I have learned that this one communicates relief. She reports that she is feeling better than last week, when she was emotionally and physically spent as a result of the hectic holiday season during which she strived to live up to extraordinarily high standards of performance as a mother, grandmother, wife, and sister: She could acknowledge that these almost inflexible standards were an ongoing source of rage. In eight years of analytic work, she has gradually been able to acknowledge that the holiday periods are especially stressful because they exacerbate chronic, relentless, internal pressure to take care of everyone's expressed, and unexpressed, need and desire. The internal pressure she feels to be the perfect caregiver generates abundant rage, making her susceptible to TMS.

She says that she is better because the holidays are finally over and she does not have to attend to so many guests and four grandchildren. (Here, I remember a dream fragment from years ago: "My handbag is overflowing. I see, tucked in a corner, a little mouse nibbling on a piece of lettuce." We had identified this as an example of how Mrs. R takes care of everyone, no matter how busy she is.) She reports that the stress is not entirely over because her oldest daughter, Pam, Pam's one-year-old daughter, and the nanny will be living in her home during the month of January. She mentions that, once again, her granddaughter's crying awakened her last night, evidencing how exquisitely attuned she is to the baby's emotional states. She can't seem not to notice, not to live on high alert, when a baby is around. We know that this intense attunement is in part related to her guilt about not being able to be there for her first-born child and, perhaps, about lingering feelings of responsibility for Alexa's accident.

Today, Mrs. R is recognizing that her daughter's living arrangement causes her great conflict: Pam has traveled back and forth from the west coast to the east coast the last year because of her employment situation, accompanied by her daughter and nanny. Mrs. R has become increasingly able to tolerate how conflicted she feels about these circumstances. Specifically, she is compelled to make Pam's life as stress-free as possible because she keenly identifies with the demands of being a mother of young children. At the same time, she is angry because she is feeling intruded upon. The presence of the nanny does little to assure Mrs. R that her granddaughter is being cared for adequately. So, with considerable simmering anger because she is giving up her freedom, she modifies her busy schedule to watch over the child. She had been feeling "so free" prior to this granddaughter's birth—so free after being a devoted mother to her four children. Here, I want to stress that grandparents are susceptible to feelings of guilt, along with abundant joy.

Mrs. R has realized that, during many years of devotion, she has also felt angry many times, "trapped" in the highly demanding role that she has always defined for herself as a sister, parent, and wife. She and I have found that her recurring musculoskeletal pains during these years were linked to these feelings that she had previously been unable to acknowledge—that is, angry feelings associated with her self-image as sister, mother, grandmother, and wife were sealed away, thus the appearance of the physical symptoms.

However, despite all of our efforts, Mrs. R has developed a skin condition since Pam and her daughter have been staying with her. It has become so severe that she must take oral cortisone medication. Today, after elaborating on this situation at home and acknowledging her chronic anger at her husband for not helping at all with household management (another major stressor), Mrs. R reports that, since our last session, she had a very sharp pain in her left foot that lasted about 24 hours. I remember, silently, that it sounded like the pain she had in her foot last spring for several months, and similar to the pain she developed after the birth of Steven. This pain prevents her from playing tennis, one of her sources of pleasure. Last year, she consulted an orthopedist who told her that the pain was due to "inflammation of unknown etiology." I mention this pain episode to Mrs. R. She says she had not thought of that pain in the current context.

After describing the recent pain, she says, "Oh, and I had a silly little dream that didn't make any sense," and quickly goes on to report that something very upsetting happened since she saw me last week. Her youngest daughter, Sarah, had received a call from the man who boards her horse, Robbie—the horse she's had since childhood. Sarah had ridden competitively as an adolescent, winning many prizes, thanks to Mrs. R's excellent instruction. The boarder said that Robbie was ill and would have to be "put down." I see that Mrs. R's eyes are tearing and her voice is breaking, slightly. She perceptibly tries to rush past experiencing this emotional response, saying impatiently, as she often does, "I don't know why I still get upset like this."

Here is a familiar decision point for me, one I've struggled with and deliberated about alone, in consultation with senior colleagues, and with Mrs. R. She has told me that she wants me to do "whatever [I] have to do" to deal with her resistance to experiencing painful feelings at times like this. I've taken various approaches.

Today, I wait. She rushes on to tell me that Sarah called her and the other family members, and they all cried and reminisced together about Robbie. She summarizes this in a couple of sentences, as I just did. We know that her "objective" way of reporting is a style that helps her distance herself from emotions that she does not want to experience fully.

Aware that she had cried easily with her children about Robbie, I wonder why she still resists crying in my presence. I have seen it as part of my job to help her connect feelings with her life experiences. Have I been too controlling, like her mother? Is that why she is resisting? On the other hand, there have been so many sessions in which I have not pursued her. Perhaps I have given her too much room to move at her own pace, afraid of being sadistic with my inquiries and priorities.

I move from this self-critical ruminating to puzzle about the 24 hours of foot pain that she mentioned in the context of Robbie's death. You can hear how intent I am on identifying the source(s) of this pain. I flash back to the dramatic relief from months of pain that she had experienced after our initial session 8 years ago. I wonder how to proceed.

I do not confront her resistance to experiencing her feelings. Instead, I inquire about the "silly" dream. After these years of working together, Mrs. R knows that I value her dreams because they have shed light on what is happening outside of consciousness. Our work on her dreams has provided "links" to significant, usually painful feelings. She becomes frustrated when she cannot readily understand them. Calling them "silly," she will humorously point her finger at me and say, "Now don't bother to get out your paper and pencil for this one!" I ask about the dream. This is the dream:

> We're [she and her husband] in a house. I know there are animals outside. I don't know what kinds. Inside, there's a mother and two puppies—Weimaraners. They need food. I'm not giving them any. Something's wrong with the puppies. They have bumps all over them. That's the dream. Very strange.

Now we begin a familiar and challenging process—I try to find meaning in this "silly" dream. I ask, "What about all these animals?" She knows that animals are important dream images because she has strong feelings for them and is especially fond of dogs. When she was growing up, her mother did not approve of dogs. As an adult she has found much pleasure in them. Currently, she has two and has lost others that we have grieved together during the treatment. She is emotionally spontaneous with her dogs and loves them because they are so directly expressive of their feelings, especially their affection. They do not resist expressing feelings—they are not embarrassed or ashamed. She loves teaching them how to obey in training classes. We have had many sessions devoted to dogs and she has had numerous dreams about them. Often, they are strays that have been abandoned or they are in cages. She rescues them.

We have painstakingly linked the theme of abandoned dogs to her anguish over feeling that she abandoned Steven. She believes that she would not have been able to take care of a child who was limited physically and intellectually because she is so threatened by feelings of dependency and vulnerability of any kind—particularly that of young infants, and of herself when she is not well physically. She feels compelled to eliminate all signs of dependency and vulnerability by "curing" them as soon as possible. These links between dogs and Steven, so salient for me, remain at an intellectual level, devoid of feelings, much of the time for Mrs. R. Their emotional significance still seems elusive to her.

I am remembering these links we have established over years of hard work and remain convinced that the dream is potentially very rich. I see, however, that Mrs. R is experiencing one of her frequent, seemingly "blank" states as she tries to associate to the animals. She maintains steady eye contact, her dark brown eyes pushing me away as she says, emphatically, "Nothing." I marvel again, silently, how impervious she can seem at times like this, times that seem so filled with meaning for me. In these all too frequent dreaded, dead spaces, tolerating my own feelings has often been difficult. Sometimes, I have felt that my head could explode at any moment.

Today, I have the sensation of "bursting at the seams with meaning and feeling," while Mrs. R exudes a wall of silence. I try to penetrate that wall by saying that we know how important animals are to her. Silence. Not to be subdued, I ask, "Why Weimarwraners?" Mrs. R says she has no idea. They are not the kind of dogs she has, however a friend, Martha, has two Weimaraners puppies and doesn't know how to take care of them—at least not the way Mrs. R would. With satisfaction, she reports that she has been trying very hard not to act on her desire to take care of everybody (remember the dream about the mouse?). This desire to take care of everybody could include telling Martha how to take care of her puppies. As a result of our work, she has decided not to offer advice to Martha, but will compromise by answering questions if Martha asks. I inquire, "What about the bumps on the puppies?" She does not know, because Weimaraners have very smooth coats. We marvel together at the smoothness and satiny sheen of their coats.

Mrs. R sits like she is carved of granite. This morning, I am challenged by her impenetrability. I struggle to stay alive in the session, to make emotional contact with her, to have an impact on her emotional state. I silently associate to the mother Weimaraner and to Martha, mothers who are not equipped to take care of their puppies. I remember that in the dream Mrs. R is, uncharacteristically, not offering food to the disfigured puppies. I mention this to her. She remains silent, unmoved.

I continue my active, vigorous pursuit of meaning—silently. I remember that Robbie, the horse that had to be put down, has been in the family for about 20 years. I muse about the time frame here, wondering aloud what was going on in the family at the time they acquired the horse. Mrs. R answers that Robbie arrived when all the kids were still at home. She reminisces about the many good times she had teaching Sarah to ride Robbie competitively. Their bond was particularly satisfying because Mrs. R had wanted to ride horses as an adolescent, but her mother did not approve of such an activity for a girl.

A bit tentatively, I remember, aloud, that that was probably about the time that Steven died. She looks stunned. I see her eyes come alive. I have touched her. We engage. She starts to elaborate on what was happening in the family in those days. Her eyes fill with tears. Wondering if I'm overreaching, I suggest a connection between her foot pain and the memory of losing Steven that might have been triggered by Robbie's death. As she weeps, she offers this interpretation: "Maybe the reason I have been so devoted to dogs and taken care of them so well for so long is because I couldn't take care of my son." I could feel my own eyes start to fill as the session ended.

I felt compelled to write detailed notes on the session immediately, in almost the same form I have just shared with you. Reflecting on the need I felt to capture this session, I realized that I had to write the process of the session to have a record that we had made such a "dramatic" connection between emotions and pain. Through hard work in therapy, together we discovered that her inability to acknowledge these feelings was related to the development of her musculoskeletal pain. My greatest challenge in the work with her was to keep feelings alive, accessible. I have slowly, but persistently, tried to help Mrs. R think about Steven and allow herself to feel about what happened to her and to Steven. Feeling the loss and the range of feelings about him helped her complete the grieving process.

Mrs. R did not repress knowledge of Steven; she remembered her first child and what happened after he was born. However, she consciously tried not to think about him because to think about him could stir up intense, undesirable feelings, such as guilt and shame. The feelings she could not tolerate having directly about Steven were experienced directly and intensely in other relationships. As I noted earlier, she was able to experience keen empathy for animals and for anyone who is in need. The unacknowledged guilt about not being able to take care of Steven, however, seemed to compel her to take care of everyone in need, no matter how much stress it caused her. This hypothesis is in line with her interpretation at the end of the session, "Maybe the reason I've been so devoted to dogs and taken care of them so well for so long is because I couldn't take care of my son."

When I met Mrs. R, she was compulsively devoted to caring for others, giving almost no consideration to her own needs. She could not permit herself to think of Steven or to feel anger at Alexa or anyone close to her. This led to a build of rage in her reservoir, spilling over into physical symptoms. In the therapy process, she was gradually able to experience feelings about losing Steven and come to feel less intense guilt about not being able to take care of him. She now has greater compassion for herself. She also found a way to acknowledge and tolerate hateful, angry feelings toward Alexa and others. This process has resulted in dramatic relief from musculoskeletal pain and allowed her to have more joy.

At the end of our second session, Mrs. R asked me,

"Will I like myself when we are finished?" At the end of this session eight years later, I think she would answer, "Yes."

[5] Spina bifida (SB) is a neural tube defect (a disorder involving incomplete development of the brain, spinal cord, and/or their protective coverings) caused by the failure of the fetus's spine to close properly during the first month of pregnancy. Infants born with SB sometimes have an open lesion on their spine where significant damage to the nerves and spinal cord has occurred. Although the spinal opening can be surgically repaired shortly after birth, the nerve damage is permanent, resulting in varying degrees of paralysis of the lower limbs. Even when there is no lesion present, there may be improperly formed or missing vertebrae and accompanying nerve damage. In addition to physical and mobility difficulties, most individuals have some form of learning disability. The three most common types of SB are: myelomeningocele, the severest form, in which the spinal cord and its protective covering (the meninges) protrude from an opening in the spine; meningocele, in which the spinal cord develops normally but the meninges protrude from a spinal opening; and occulta, the mildest form, in which one or more vertebrae are malformed and covered by a layer of skin. SB may also cause bowel and bladder complications, and many children with SB have hydrocephalus (excessive accumulation of cerebrospinal fluid in the brain). (www.ninds.nih.gov/disorders/spina_bifida/spina_bifida)

Little Kate's Journey

Kate, age 40, came for a focused consultation 6 months after having met Dr. Sarno, who gave her a diagnosis of TMS. By the time we met, she was pain-free most of the time, but she wanted additional help to reduce the pain even further. She was living abroad for the past year because her husband had received a business promotion, which required them to relocate to a distant city in Asia. Despite severe back pain, Kate, highly responsible and competent since early childhood, had relocated their household and two children, an eight-year-old daughter and a three-year-old son, a year before we met.

In preparation for 5 sessions within a 4 day period, I asked Kate to send me all background information that she thought would be helpful to us as I prepared to give her the help she was seeking.

She gave her history of back pain as follows:

> Since the age of 26, I've desperately searched for a cure to my back pain, always hopeful and optimistic that each practitioner I visited would be the one to correct my back problem and give me back my life. I've spent thousands and thousands of dollars, plus wasted hundreds of hours going to chiropractors, sport clinics, physiotherapy, osteopaths in a desperate attempt, religiously following, to the book, every stretch, exercise and ointment they ever gave me. I've tried every available alternative therapy plus mainstream medicine searching for a cure for my mystery back problem. Over the past 15 years this has taken its toll on the people who are close to me as well as myself. I remember all the holidays

that have been ruined, all the special occasions
where the fear and conditioning that goes with this
has controlled my life, all the enjoyment I received
from my passion for exercise and sport plus the love
and involvement I had with my kids was taken away
from me. I've been consumed with my back for
most of my adult life and up until I saw Dr. Sarno
last January.

In the journal entries she sent me regarding the sources of her TMS, Kate described her early childhood and young adulthood poignantly, in a manner that would evoke empathy and compassion in most readers, and particularly in those of us familiar with triggers for TMS.

Childhood

The first nine years of my childhood were very
happy and normal. From nine onwards, I can
remember my Mother becoming very depressed
and looked to religion for help. This coincided
with Mom having a hysterectomy. When I was
12, my Mother attempted to take her life, which
went terribly wrong and left her disabled in both
of her hands: She tried to cut her wrists. My Father
recently described this as a cry for help, which went
tragically wrong!

The next three years my carefree childhood ended,
I remember various incidences where my Mother
tried to take her life again.
According to my Father, she was attempting to
escape from the pain of her disability, which sadly
was a constant reminder of what she did to herself!

One particular incident sticks in my mind. After returning from school, I found her lying in bed with plastic bags wrapped tightly over her head, secured with elastic bands.

Our lives during this period evolved around my Mother's moods—her good days and bad days! We would dread coming home from school, scared to find what state she would be in.

At the age of 16, I remember my Father picking us up from school and telling us the tragic news about Mom's death. I never knew exact details of how she died until six weeks ago, when I confronted my Father and asked him. I was always wary of bringing the subject up before as my Father has been through so much and I didn't want to upset him. My Father told me my Mother's heart simply stopped beating: He said she gave up the will to live! This breaks my heart, as she left behind three children who adored and needed their mother.

As a Mother, I find this so hard to comprehend: How could a mother ever want to leave behind her children, completely innocent victims, to fend for themselves in such a completely selfish act and waste of a life? I feel so angry and disappointed with her, although I'm happier knowing that she did actually die naturally rather than kill herself, despite the fact she wanted to kill herself. She died of a broken heart because of the physical mess due to her own foolish attempt on her life.

I don't think I've ever forgiven my Mother for what she did. I pity her but I can't forgive her. With my own children, I have a very strong desire to be the mother I never had. I would never put my children through what my mother put me through. Although I have considered suicide when my back pain was at its worst, I've always snapped out of my self-pity and put my children first.

Shortly after my Mother died, my Grandfather died of a tumor, and then two years later my grandmother took her own life. I think she never came to terms with losing her daughter, and then her husband. She was the closet person we had next to our Mother and Father. It broke all of our hearts to try and understand why she wanted to leave us behind just like Mom did!

Early adulthood

At 21, a capable, ambitious young woman who valued physical fitness, Kate developed a health club with two partners. Working very hard—"I had tremendous drive" — the first two years were very successful.

Shortly after this, my Nana died, and we started to experience financial problems due to high bank interest rates. This was around the time when I first experienced my first episode of tremendous back pain.

Despite the pain and depression, Kate taught four to five fitness classes each day, in addition to sessions with personal training clients. Her strong sense of responsibility and integrity kept her going:

> I had no choice but continue teaching classes
> despite the chronic pain I was in with my back and
> the depression this brought. I had to work. This was
> my business. I had to honor my financial debt to
> the bank and my parents, as they had secured our
> financial debt to the bank by acting as guarantors.

Reflecting in her journal on this review of her childhood and young adulthood, she wrote:

I look back now and I really don't know how I managed. My life consisted of chronic back pain, trying to teach step aerobic classes, the financial stress of making a business work, the emotional stress of my business partners and my family, plus my own unhappy love life.

Marriage and Children

Kate met her husband, Rick, through mutual friends. After three years together, they married when Kate was 32. They conceived their daughter, Anna, very quickly. Waiting three weeks for the Downs syndrome screening test results "was one of the worst times of my life...I was an emotional mess, my body almost shut down, my back went, I had an eye infection, and just couldn't stop crying." She delivered a "beautiful healthy baby girl." Both she and her husband we eager to have a large family, so they tried to conceive a year later. After trying for a year, she got pregnant but had a miscarriage after 12 weeks: "We were devastated." After going on a "mission" to get pregnant, she had two miscarriages and two failed IVF procedures. They decided to stop trying: "Our marriage was suffering and we simply couldn't go through the agony of another miscarriage. I was told at the age of 37 I was biologically too old to have another baby, and if I did naturally conceive the outcome would most definitely be a miscarriage." Living with broken hearts at this pronouncement, nevertheless they conceived naturally. "I was petrified from beginning to end. I look at him today and he's my little miracle. I'm the luckiest Mother...against all the odds." Kate went through this prolonged, acutely stressful period with a "bad back," pressing on despite her pain.

In her pre-consultation journal and in our focused consultation, Kate identified her relationship with her husband as another stressor. When they met, she "fell for him straight away." She loved his "boyish quality of enjoying life" but has discovered that "this sometimes infuriates me, as I often feel his enjoyment for life encroaches on family time with the children." Rick, also a hard worker, is strongly committed to support his family financially. The tension points in their marriage are around their different views of how to raise their children:

> Most of our arguments are to do with the children as we have different views on bringing up the children. He is more laid back and I think pretty selfish, whereas due to my own unhappy childhood I'm very much more hands on, wanting to spend as much quality time with the kids as possible.

Our consultation focused on Kate's overwhelming childhood experiences, significant losses in early adulthood, and the stresses and pleasures of marriage and parenting. In her journaling, she had developed some "cognitive" appreciation for just how difficult life had been and how these difficult experiences became triggers for back pain that became chronic. What I felt Kate needed was to experience a keener emotional, or feeling, connection with the enormity of the impact of the numerous acute and chronic stresses she had endured and survived, even thrived. Near the end of the fourth session, the day before she was scheduled to return to Asia, I gently inquired, "I wonder what little Kate has been feeling throughout these challenging times?" Kate seemed a little surprised by my question: She thought she had experienced most of what she needed to experience, based on how rapidly her back pain had resolved. Knowing her tenacity, I expected that she would ponder this carefully until we had our last session the next day.

As we began our last session, I wondered what would evolve, and I felt sad that she was leaving for a distant city with so few supports available to her there. Even though we had arranged to have phone/video consultations to follow up, I was wishing we could continue our work in person. She began by telling me that she'd had a big fight with her husband last night over her needing a certain kind of attention from him that she felt he hadn't given. After the fight, she locked herself in the bathroom and cried for the first time in many years. She was crying for "little Kate." She spoke, with great feeling, about her realization of just what "little Kate" had endured. Together, we made a plan for the many ways in which she could take care of "little Kate" now.

About a week after her return to Asia, she sent me her journal entry about her last appointment with me. Her words say it far more evocatively than I ever could:

> I went to my appointment today feeling very tense and emotional. This morning while writing my notes, I went to the bathroom and wept uncontrollably for how I was feeling inside. I wept for the child inside me, "little Kate," the child who at the age of nine started to lose her childhood, following the onset of Mom's depression and

eventually her attempted suicide and death. This child remains deep within—frightened, abandoned, insecure, introverted, desperately looking for her Mother's love. I realize that being married to Rick creates tension for little Kate, as there are times when she feels she carries the burden and responsibility—this time for her children not her mother. I need to learn to nurture little Kate, mother her as I would mother my own children. Her personality is sensitive similar to my daughter's. I need to predict how she is feeling during uncomfortable moments of confrontation and how she deals with times of sadness and anger. The child is immature and in constant conflict with the Kate of today. I need to write about little Kate and relate it to daily situations. I need to relate little Kate to my feeling towards Rick and how he sometimes makes me feel.

The advice Fran gave me.
I need to:
1. Treat the inner child, little Kate, the way I would treat my own. Understand how she is feeling, understand her immature personality, a young child's personality, who from the age of nine lost her childhood. Her resentment, her selfishness, her sensitivity, and her insecurities in relationships.
2. I need to learn to be more direct and assertive with Rick, to say no when I don't want to do something, rather than letting little Kate make the decision and then confronting this decision later on. This makes him very angry and confused as I keep changing my mind. I need to be more assertive

in the beginning, and I need to let him know I'm going to behave this way.
- joint responsibility for children
- joint responsibility for holidays and leisure time
- communication of how I'm feeling and little Kate is feeling during confrontation and arguments.

3. To do a list of day-to-day chores of a Mother and show Rick so he understands what I do.
4. To write in my journal every day, helping little Kate relate to marriage with Rick.
5. Keep asking myself /little Kate—How do I feel?

I will have online sessions by phone. Also e-mail notes for Fran to read, to see if I'm on the right track.

It's important for little Kate to grieve for her loss. When I wept in the bathroom back in New York, I was weeping for the loss of my mother.

The Legacy of Harsh Parenting
Mr. L and the Tenacious Inner Critic

Three days after he was examined by Dr. Sarno and given the TMS diagnosis, Mr. L, age 64, shed the back brace he had worn every day for 25 years. Mr. L had had back surgery about 20 years earlier to repair a herniated disc. He recovered from the surgery and returned to a very active lifestyle that involved a hectic travel schedule in order to run his very successful business. He had worn the corset all those years because he was terrified that he would injure himself without it.

Mr. L started individual psychotherapy on a once-a-week schedule five months after receiving a TMS diagnosis in October 2006. One of the facts that he told me in our first session was that his father, who died in 1993, had informed him when he was age 18 that he was a bigamist. In fact, he had another family living nearby that included a son. Their relationship, always problematic, became even more strained thereafter—so much so that Mr. L did not speak to his father in the 25-30 years before he died. He banished him from his life. In the first half year of therapy, Mr. L gave examples of how competitive his father had been with him and his brother, five years younger. His father consistently, ruthlessly made him feel like a failure if he noticed him, or like he didn't exist at all. As I listened, I could easily sense the impact of his father's narcissism on Mr. L's self-esteem. It took several months for me to find a way to bring this to Mr. L's attention without injuring him further. I will use a session from spring 2007 to illustrate how I brought this to his attention and how we related it to his TMS symptoms.

Mr. L and I resume our weekly meeting schedule after a 4-week break when I was on vacation, then he was on vacation, and then I was sick. This unanticipated disruption was unfortunate because we had recently begun to help him hear how harsh and critical he can be toward himself when he doesn't measure up to his very high standards. If

Mr. L gave you details about his track record, you would be astounded to hear him call himself a "failure" in life. Further, he calls himself "stupid" because he feels like a failure.

Mr. L is a presence to be reckoned with. Soon to be 65, he is athletic, trim, and dresses in an understated, youthful style. His white hair frames chiseled features and piercing blue eyes. His trenchant dissection of any topic, sarcastic sense of humor, and resonant voice have kept me on my toes in our sessions. He takes our work very seriously. Mulling between sessions, he tries to use what we've discussed, engaging me easily at the beginning of each session with an update. Our interchanges are often fun because I enjoy his sense of humor, but he rarely laughs. Unsmiling, his craggy face could be intimidating and keep people at a distance. In a breakthrough session a couple of months ago, when I gently made this observation, he was stunned. He had no idea what I was talking about. In subsequent sessions, I brought it to his attention when I noticed it. In the following vignette from today's session, I will illustrate how we increased Mr. L's awareness of the ways in which he had unconsciously adopted his father's harsh parenting attitude toward himself. In doing so, he was constantly creating more unconscious rage at being treated badly, by himself. Over many years, this had led to a reservoir of rage that could overflow at any time. It was no surprise that he had been plagued by TMS symptoms during these years.

Mr. L began the session by telling me that he had been doing fine, pain-free for almost three months now. Monday night of the previous week, the old pain in his leg returned, just after he had arrived home in Manhattan. He was furious and disappointed. He just couldn't figure it out, and this constituted more evidence that he is a failure in life. Feeling like a failure made him feel stupid and angry at himself. I responded by inquiring about the events during the weeks we had not had sessions. His response was that everything had been fine while he was away for a few weeks in his vacation home and then he'd had an excellent traveling vacation with good friends. "I was fine until I got home Monday night." Remembering previous discussions about how he feels about his retirement life in Manhattan, I asked, "How did you feel about being home?" He responded, "I'm bored."

I lead him in an exploration of why he's bored, which we've discussed in previous sessions. He's bored even though he has several interests that he pursues on a regular basis, but that's not enough to justify his existence. What does he have to complain about—he has few problems, an easy life. I remind him that we discovered a couple of months ago that he can be free of pain while he's out of state in his vacation home: It's legitimate to be having leisure and pleasure in that location. His internal critic does not permit that in Manhattan, it seems.

He remembers our having worked on this and quickly critiques his failure to have remembered it sooner. I notice the expression on his face, his eyes cold like an eagle moving in to attack its chosen prey. His voice is harsh. I visibly wince and ask, "I wonder what it's like for you inside when you evaluate yourself that way?" At first he doesn't know what I'm referring to. I spell it out for him. He says, "I really don't hear the tone of my voice." I try to replicate it for him. He still doesn't hear it. I suggest that he start noticing it throughout the day. Then I remind him that we know where he learned this: He recalls that we had discussed that he treats himself the way his father treated him.

On September 10, 2008, Mr. L reports the following:
> The intellectual understanding—that your TMS is caused by the overflowing of the "reservoir of rage" —is not the most difficult achievement of your TMS journey. The hard part is accepting that, whatever the circumstances that have brought you to this point, your TMS is, in large part, due to the idea that "you are not happy with yourself and that you are not accepting of yourself." This is, for me, the area in which psychotherapy has been most helpful in the battle against TMS and myself. It is the recognition that I don't have to be in a "battle" with myself, that I can allow myself to be more satisfied with myself, and that seems to, in some way, keep the "reservoir of rage" from overflowing as often as it used to.

Self-Sufficient, Too Early
Ms. T

Ms. T came for an initial consultation about one month after her 80th birthday. For this discussion, she asked that I describe her as married, the mother of 6, and after a variety of jobs then became the Executive Director and then President of a New York City foundation for the last 30 years. Writing to me in 2008, she reiterated the medical history she gave me in that consultation:

> My adventure with TMS began about four years ago, shortly after I had received a diagnosis of

colon cancer, for which I had the required surgery and recovered quite quickly. Eight months later I developed what was described as a "dropped foot." I couldn't hold my left foot up, causing me to trip a lot. Following a visit to a neurosurgeon, I submitted to the operation he recommended, a laminectomy. I had lumber stenosis, he said, causing pressure on the sciatic nerve and pain and some numbness on the outside of my lower left leg. The operation was urgent, he said. My recovery was uneventful. Before too long, however, I began suffering intermittent but excruciating pain in my left buttock. It was interfering with my life and showed no signs of abating. I consulted another neurosurgeon, the earlier one having retired. The new doctor was a delightful young man who had studied the mandatory MRI required before an appointment could be made. He reported that I had a herniated disc, and so on. His take on my problem was grim. He recommended spinal fusion and various titanium implants. He added that my age, 79, put me in the high risk category. Furthermore, he could not guarantee results as far as pain reduction was concerned. Perhaps one could hope for a 50% improvement, he said. My husband of 36 years, who had accompanied me, and I thanked the doctor and departed, saying that we needed to think about what he had told us.

Ms. T's primary care physician recommended Dr. Sarno's books, which she read, and saw him in early June of 2005:
We met, talked, and he examined me, giving me

the diagnosis TMS. He told me that previous
alarming diagnoses from neurosurgeons were
to be set aside. The cause of my pain was acute
unconscious feelings of repressed anger. He went
on to draw me a picture of a "reservoir," as he
called it, explaining that the first third of it was
filled with childhood hurts and disappointments.
The second third was filled with anger and dismay
at the vicissitudes of life. In my case, it was now
overflowing with the shock of the recent cancer
diagnosis and the concomitant fear of aging
and mortality. Dr. Sarno emphasized that the
unconscious is childish and timeless and the angers,
hurts, and rages of a lifetime are cumulative.

Ms. T attended his lectures and small groups, and did his home-study writing program:

Despite my diligence, the debilitating pain
continued. I was unable to walk down a city block
without frequent stops to allow the pain to subside.
Often I held onto the side of buildings to support
myself. Pain killers offered no relief, adding
to my conviction that my problem was indeed
psychological not physical.
After several weeks of reporting no improvement
in my condition at one of the small group sessions,
Dr. Sarno suggested psychotherapy.
I entered the process with the strong conviction
that an essential element would be that the client
and therapist be a good match. What I found
difficult, in the beginning, was overcoming feelings
of intense loyalty to members of my family who
had unwittingly caused me pain in my childhood.

It took time and a great deal of help to realize
that my parents did the best they could given
their parenting limitations and what mattered
and needed to be explored were the feelings their
actions evoked in me. Dr. Anderson's searching
questions led me to focus on situations that surely
engendered sadness, anger, and rage. It took us
many weeks to come to grips with the fact that I
had suffered from inordinate benign neglect when I
was little.

Based on her understanding of TMS when I met her, Ms. T stated, "I fit the profile: high expectations and low self-confidence; perfectionistic; need to be liked. I have a stiff upper lip—I don't show my emotions." In her home-study writing, she had connected her longstanding fear of being a passenger in a car to an accident when riding in a taxi with her governess:
At age six, a front tooth was knocked out in a
taxi collision resulting in my having to wear a
false tooth on a retainer until I was 18, when
a permanent device could be installed. I was
embarrassed throughout my childhood and fearful
that my false tooth would be discovered.
She had multiple bones broken in her face. She returned home from the hospital but soon her mother went out to a dinner engagement, leaving the governess to take care of her. "There was a pattern of nobody being there. Neither of my parents was there to offer comfort. My care was in the hands of others."

Praise for accomplishments in school or in sports
and the like was absent. Criticism for anything less

than excellent performance prevailed. "Unflattering
comments were made about my appearance. In
those days, saying anything positive was seen as
'spoiling' children."

Another memory of "nobody being there" was when she
fell on the ice and injured her left thigh:
I was doing a solo figure skating program. I fell
because there was a bobby pin on the ice, which
stopped me abruptly, causing a fall. The fall resulted
in the back of my right blade penetrating my left
thigh, causing a deep wound and profuse bleeding. I
was about 12 years old.
This time the family's chauffeur was the one who
oversaw medical treatment, as best she could remember.

Another childhood memory, age uncertain, depicted
how skilled she was at not showing her feelings. She
recalled sitting on her father's lap and feeling his cigarette
burning her left leg, "But I didn't move."

Her parents divorced when she was six. Ms. T and her
brother, 13 months older, supported their alcoholic father as
he aged.

"I married at 19 and wanted to be the world's best
mother." She had four children right away, and divorced
after eight years. She had two more children with her second
husband before they divorced after 13 years.

At the end of our first session, she said, "I hurt less
coming to you."

Ms. T began our second session by reporting three
dreams since we met. In the first dream, she was at a dance
rehearsal witnessing a dog chasing a horse, whose leg was
tied to the floor. In the dream, she felt frustrated because she

couldn't help the horse. This took us into a discussion about how important it is to her to feel that she can help others. It's very difficult for her to tolerate feeling helpless. She associated to her mother's death six years earlier: "I took care of her for the last five months of her life. I felt helpless because she didn't like receiving help."

At the beginning of our third session, she reported, "I feel the pain is less." She went on to speak about sensing the "drumbeat of death," acknowledging her fear of aging and mortality. She noted that she was near the second anniversary of her colon cancer surgery and fears that it will recur. She remembered that her maternal grandfather died when she was five or six, and rather than attending the funeral, "my brother and I were sent away." Her maternal grandmother died one year later.

> Both of my maternal grandparents died within a year when I was about five years old. My parents divorced shortly thereafter. My father was an alcoholic and my mother soon had a demanding career. Dr. Anderson told me that a mother's attention is lifeblood, an essential nutrient for a small child. My mother's attention had been limited, probably causing me to repress emotions. I began to understand that independence had been thrust upon me at a very early age.

The theme of experiencing numerous losses continued: Her brother lost two wives at untimely ages. "I realize that I've had an inordinate number of experiences with death: three of my close business associates were killed in accidents." She encountered another kind of loss after her colon surgery: She had chronic diarrhea for one and a half to two years, which severely restricted her freedom to keep up her active schedule: "I'm not good at sitting still."

In the fourth session, she reported, "I'm walking more. I don't have to stop to rest as often. I'm less of a perfectionist."

She opens the sixth session, having reflected on the theme of rushing as a source of TMS pain, "I have spent most of my life rushing. Rushing generated anger. I get resentful." She then gave some examples of noticing that she was rushing and how the rushing generated internal pressure in planning the details of several social events. "I've always taken on too much. I've always had a high-pressure job. I've sought out pressure. I have to finish every book I start, even if I don't like it." These observations take her to a realization that "I don't like having help. I'm a one-man band. The pain has slowed me up."

Six weeks into the treatment she reports longer periods with no pain, and "I can walk pain-free." Ms. T registers at her gym, a vote of confidence that she will resume her athletics. I learned more about the importance of being self-sufficient, physically autonomous: Ms. T started ice skating at 8 years of age and flying at age 15. "My main feeling was independence," which her mother allowed, but she drew the line when Ms. T wanted to be a fashion model. Her low self-esteem about her appearance was triggered in part by feedback from her father when she was an emerging adolescent: "I had a hang-up about not being attractive. My father had pictures of great beauties he had dated in his apartment. My father told me I was too tall and too flat-chested. He thought that my brother was special and that I was intelligent."

Around this time, Ms. T mentioned that she "moved a great deal" when she was growing up and gave several examples. Three weeks later, at my suggestion, she made a list of the residences that she could remember. Both of us were surprised that between birth and age 19, when she married, she had lived in nine residences in New York City and four others outside the city:

> I had been aware of difficulties in my childhood but not my feelings about them. In therapy, we looked at other circumstances that troubled me in my early years. For instance, Dr. Anderson asked me where "home" was as I was growing up. Well, I reported, we moved a lot, maybe every couple of years. She asked me to bring a list of all the addresses I remembered. The exercise of making that list made me realize how disturbing and unsettling the lack of a permanent home surely was to me, and that I had stifled those feelings and so many others.

At the beginning of this three-week period, Ms. T had a dream in which her father was holding a baby: "A disaster. His wife had died. He leaned over and dropped the baby." I asked how she felt in the dream: "I felt scared for the baby. I woke up concerned." Her associations led us to some positive memories of being with her father and brother. Something about the dreamed reminded her of a scene from a photo of them on the beach. "It all ended when I was seven or eight," shortly after her parents divorced.

More associations rushed in, bringing memories of being lonely as a child. Ms. T was the second child of a highly successful mother, who defied any stereotype about the married woman from that era. Highly engaged in business that required many hours away from home, Ms. T and her brother were cared for by governesses, housekeepers, and chauffeurs. She was able to remember one of her mother's trips to Europe when her father's sister looked in on them: "I cried and said, 'You're not my mommy.'"

I asked how she comforted herself during these times.

As a young child, self-comfort was sucking her fingers, until the first accident. "As an adolescent, I went out to La Guardia to watch the planes." Exploring her interest in learning to fly, she puzzled, "How far would I have to go for you to stop me? I was in control flying compared with being in the car accident." She had a hidden agenda in learning to fly: "I wanted to be in the Women's Air Transport, but I was too young. I was aware of the war."

In the next session, she said she had walked 20 blocks without pain for the first time. She was becoming even more aware of feeling rushed and she doesn't like it. Near the end of this session, she gave the following summary of what we had discovered after 10 weeks of psychotherapy: 1) I didn't have a home; 2) I was emotionally neglected; 3) My mother had her own problems.

(1/26/06) In a discussion of several dreams, the "tidy theme" emerged, one manifestation of perfectionism that can cause stress and TMS symptoms. There are other dream details that remind her of numbers of people she has lost:

> In addition to the premature deaths of two grandparents, my brother's first wife died at the age of 21 when I was 19. A subsequent wife of my brother's died suddenly from a brain aneurism at the age of 40. She and I were close friends and about the same age. My father died shortly afterwards. Through our discussions, I came to understand how this pattern of deaths affects me as I confront aging and mortality. Dr. Anderson recommended that I read *How We Die* by Dr. Newland and *The Life Cycle Completed* by Eric Erikson to better understand the various stages of life and to become less fearful of the process.

One association was to the untimely death of a friend due to cancer. For the first time, Ms. T directly links her TMS pain with fears about her cancer returning: "Every time the pain came up I thought about cancer."

(1/31/06) "I have noticed less and less pain." The dream theme of "cleaning up" emerges, a variation on "tidying." She refers to it as her compulsive behavior. We discuss mixed feelings towards people she loves. This makes her feel freer of her mother's approval.

Two sessions later, the pain on her right side is worse, and I recommend that she speak with Dr. S. We explore possible reasons for the pain, and she realizes the pressure she's feeling about the strained and unhappy relationship with her younger half-sister and that it caused her anger and pain. She has a dream that yields the theme of trying to "glue" something together that couldn't possibly be done. She has to deal with her half-sister, Leigh, and is trying to keep a sense of humor without repressing the fact that she's still angry at her.

In the next session, she says that she spoke with Dr. Sarno about the pain in her right side. He recommends stopping the workout at the gym for a while. As we discuss her attitude while she's working out, she recognizes that it's her attitude toward the workout that is probably causing the pain: "I put pressure on myself during the workout. Maybe I'm resentful of the responsibility I've had for Leigh since she was born. It's always been a one-way street with her."

(4/4/06) She has her first dream about a little girl: "I'm holding a little girl, two and a half years old, in my arms." She remembers feeling guilty that she had left her young children to do important volunteer work. "But I wouldn't leave a two-and-a-half-year-old girl." Referring to her mother's many travels when she was young, "Mother always took us with her but we didn't always stay with her. She was not doing to us what was done to her [referring to her mother having been left with caregivers when she was young]."

(4/13/06) More discussion about overcoming fear. "I had no fear of flying. I had training in hiding my feelings. No one is as careful as I am." (5/2/06) "I don't like anyone to see me vulnerable." (5/4/06) Pain is diminishing greatly. (5/11/06) Had a good week last week. Going to the gym two times a week. (5/16/06) The TMS pain is almost gone. "I had a dream in which a mother is not concerned in the least about her children, ages one to six, who are jumping around." I point out that the mother is not concerned. She responds, "I'm the worrier."

(6/22/06) At the beginning of several weeks at her vacation home: "I feel guilty that I haven't invited any of the kids to visit."

(6/28/06) A dream: "I had a baby girl, six months old. I was holding her in my arms. She was wearing a long coat I had knitted for her. I realized she needed a bottle and I didn't have one. I felt bad. I'm a worrier." Ms. T will try skating the next week for the first time since before the surgery, two years off the ice. "I'm not feeling pressured, I'm not rushing. I'm accepting that I'm not in pain. I'm accepting the aging process better."

(7/13/06) She has been on the ice four times, although she hasn't skated full sessions yet. She's had a dream in which she's on the ice and everything is normal except towards the end of a 50-minute session when she notices that people are leaving head first through an ice tunnel: "Diving head first into the unknown. I was worried that the ice might collapse. I have been thinking how I'll feel if I don't get back to where I was. I'm not good at being dependent. Being free is the great thing about skating."

In summarizing the process of psychotherapy that resulted in freedom from TMS pain, Ms. T wrote as follows:

> Gradually, my pain diminished and eventually stopped. I was able to walk in comfort enjoying this wonderful city once again. I even resumed ice dancing, a sport I very much enjoy. It seemed time to end my 12 months of therapy. I exacted assurance from Dr. Anderson that should I feel the need for further help, she would be available to me.
>
> I had learned to more effectively handle various problems in my life. Woven into our conversations were ways to handle troubling family crises. I learned how to better avoid stress and the inevitable pressures one faces as a parent, stepparent and grandparent of a very large family, and in my work. She showed me how angry feelings need not mean an absence of love, even suggesting that I simply say "no" when too much is piled on me. A daring concept for someone who wants very much to be loved, but it works! I now know that the pain was a substitute for feelings, a distraction, and that it can occur on anniversaries of traumatic events.
>
> I am able, now, to stop and think about how I feel in situations that arise, rather than plunging in head first, always so anxious to please. Hardly a day passes that I don't think of various approaches we have discussed having to do with stress management. We live busy lives in a frenetic city with constant demands made on us. It is glorious to feel inner peace and to be free of the overwhelming pain that dogged my steps for a protracted period of time.

Speaking Up for Myself
Mr. A

At the end of our first session in early November, Mr. A expressed surprise that he had talked so much about his stress at home with his wife and only child, a dearly-loved daughter, age 16. Near the beginning of the session, we began trying to identify emotional triggers related to the pain in his left shoulder that had begun before Christmas last year. He had had a year of foot, ankle, and knee pain the preceding year. Having seen Dr. Sarno for a consultation and diagnosis of TMS in early August of this year, he had been trying to identify what was making him angry, along the lines Sarno had suggested.

As he began to tell me about his marriage of 17 years and his daughter, he said, "I can't articulate when I'm angry," and gave me a recent example of a conflict with his wife in which he knew he was angry with her because "I feel like I have to shoulder too much of the responsibility around the house." This had been a problem throughout his marriage. Furthermore, he often felt they weren't "on the same page" about how to deal with their daughter, who sounded like she was behaving in expectable challenging ways for a 16-year-old. He said, "My daughter and I used to be thick as thieves" until she was around 10 years old. He said he would like to be closer to her and that he guessed that his wife might feel that he doesn't care for her because their physical intimacy had decreased drastically shortly after their daughter was born. I'm making notes as we speak and silently placing red flags on this domestic territory. He told me a bit more about their early relationship, how they had lived together three years and had a great time. He wasn't ready to get married, but his wife became pregnant and he felt that marrying her was the right thing to do. And he did, one and a half months later.

He spoke about his wife's conflict with her siblings. He comes from an Irish Catholic family of nine kids. His brother, three years older, died suddenly of cardiac failure at the age of 39. That brother was "all about having fun." His father died four years later; his mother died seven years later. Throughout these amassed losses, he felt his wife wasn't there for him.

He was the third child: "I was wedged between two athletic brothers, two successful males." He doesn't feel that he's doing as well as he would like professionally even though his income is good. "Am I not speaking up for myself?" he queries. He works freelance in the technology field and is focused on making a good income to support his family so he has to cut back on his hobbies, which is another source of stress and anger. As we conclude the session, he says he feels "better getting things off my chest," notes his surprise that he had talked so much about his home life, and says he is struck by how often he's not "speaking up for myself." We agree to meet once a week to see if our work can make an impact on his pain.

In the second session, he begins by saying that he's sleeping better. I asked for reactions to our first session. He says, "I was very surprised at the time I spent talking about domestic conflicts." I asked for recent incidents. He gave me one from early that morning. Referring to his wife, "She dismissed my opinion. She didn't listen to me. I'm angry at her and disappointed. I'm angry at myself for participating the way I did. I don't stand up for myself." He goes on to say that they never resolve this kind of conflict. "She stomps off.

We either deal with things right away or not at all." They've stopped doing things they used to enjoy, and he doesn't know why.

In the third session, he reports that his left shoulder still hurts. I suggest that he speak with Dr. Sarno. Switching to focus on emotional fuel for the pain, he said that a half hour after our last session, he realized that he felt that his wife had usurped his role. "I felt less masculine. I feel like I need to stand my ground. I feel like when I wake at night in pain, I'm clenching my left arm and shoulder. Like I'm holding back a punch. I've held back a lot." There was one night in the past week when he did speak up to his wife and had a "gloated feeling that she kind of backed down." He's surprised by his power. He also had spoken to his daughter about how he had reacted to her "rebellious" announcement that she was dyeing her hair a color he thought was outrageous. I asked him what he was like at 16 and was surprised to hear the he was the first in his family to rebel against Vietnam.

Themes that emerge: I don't have camaraderie at work (11/26/03). He brings in dreams of boys, age 7 and 10, who are very attuned to what's happening in the adult world, taking too much responsibility for adult matters. He says this is a familiar thing. There's an easy way or a hard way. He no longer wants to be doing things the hard way because he doesn't feel as invulnerable as he used to. This concerns him. "What happened to my bravado, the sense that I can do anything, even if it's crazy?"

In the fifth session (12/3/03), he reports that, after consulting with Dr. Sarno, he had an MRI of his shoulder the day before our session. Then, we go into more detail about the emotional circumstances surrounding the beginning of his left shoulder pain before Christmas last year. It was the first year that his daughter was not interested in getting a Christmas tree, a project they had always enjoyed. Rather, "she wanted to punch holes in our things," referring to how his daughter seemed to want to continue to dissolve their close relationship. He had begun to feel rejected by her, going back to two summers ago when they had taken a trip together and she had "set up a distance." "I treated my parents the same way. I feel guilty." He speaks about how low his confidence was in high school, living in his older brother's "shadow." He started to feel much better about himself in college: "It took a long time to get to be my own person."

While in college, he had a significant romantic relationship that led to an engagement. He described her as a "take charge person" who broke the engagement because he wasn't ready for responsibility. When his fiancée broke off the engagement when he was 26, he moved back in with his parents. He developed prostatitis. "I got physical symptoms: prostatitis and my irritable bowel symptoms from teenage years returned. I'd become emotionally dependent on her. I felt a need for somebody in my life." At the end of this session, we underscore the themes of lack of self-confidence and low self-esteem, together placing red flags on this territory as a major source of repressed rage that was probably associated with the development of his physical symptoms in college, and most recently in TMS shoulder pain.

In the next session (12/10/03), he reported that the MRI results could not account for the nature and severity of his shoulder pain. This outcome helped him to have confidence that addressing emotional issues could help eliminate his pain. He went on to tell me how his "stronger, dominant older brother picked on me physically and teased me, threatening to choke me." He had had dinner on the weekend with his younger sister, on the anniversary of his mother's death. He felt sad, a loss of innocence. "I feel like a ping pong ball going back and forth between home and my job. I feel disappointment about life not turning out the way I wanted." He spoke soulfully about not having made a "home" with his family and how he's jealous of his siblings who "seem to have created a wonderful life with their families." Here again, Mr. A is revealing his low self-esteem and critical self-evaluation, which provide ample fuel for TMS symptoms.

We began to identify interpersonal stressors at work. Mr. A works in solitude most of the time. A co-worker, Joe, whom he's known more than 10 years, has been working the same shift for the past year. Mr. A has ambivalent feelings about Joe, who's very outgoing and loud, in contrast with his own quiet, sarcastic sense of humor. He finds that he ends up going out to lunch with Joe, even when he doesn't want to. In fact, it's hard for him to acknowledge to himself and to me that he doesn't want to. He feels that he *should* want to. In this discussion, Mr. A interweaves a history of health problems during the past year: high blood sugar and an attack of gout in the spring (hadn't had one in more than 10 years). We wonder if internal pressure to do what the other person wants is contributing to his health problems. (12/23/03)

(1/14/04) By mid-January, he is sleeping some nights without pain: "I feel I'm back on track." We continue our discussion of how he can establish boundaries with Joe at the office, and he's trying to assert himself but it's difficult. He associates to all of the loved ones he lost within a short period and how numb he felt then and now. He can't cry, even at his mother's funeral, because her death was a relief for her and the family after her long struggle with cancer. He said, "My mother sacrificed herself for the good of others and would put anybody else's need before her." He realizes that he often behaves the same way. It's had a negative impact on his career: He feels bad about himself because he's always been on "the second string" in work situations.

(1/21/04) Consistently, he is feeling a trace more mobility in his left shoulder. Sleeping without Ambien. More pain last night. (What stressors?) Worked two long days but good news about my job—I'll be shifting to new technology. I've been writing more, per Dr. Sarno's instructions, and have discovered that I'm a "goodist." That discovery had prompted him to think about his five younger siblings and himself, reporting that "All of us are very responsible." He feels guilty that he bullied one of his younger brothers and teased a younger sister. He compared himself unfavorably with the two brothers he was "wedged in between." In contrast to Mr. A, they were very good athletes: "I was a sickly kid. I had seasonal allergies and skin problems. I always had a stomach problem. My mother worried about that." Going further, he offered, "I was sensitive, my feelings were easily hurt." His father, a very successful, high-profile professional, couldn't "nurture" Mr. A's interest in music and the arts. High school was particularly difficult because he felt so "different," so inept. In college, finally away from his family of origin and on his own, he began to feel self-confident and have fun: His symptoms went away.

By the end of January, Mr. A reports that he's made "a definite separation" from Joe. He can sense Joe's hurt feelings. Joe thinks they are "fast-buddies." He doesn't like to hurt Joe's feelings, but he just can't pretend any longer.

Soon, we begin to discuss his guilty feelings about pursuing, somewhat clandestinely, his musical interests, referring to his music as his "daily vacation." He has wondered if playing his music caused an increase in his shoulder pain. His wife isn't interested in his music, and he's afraid that she thinks he spends too much time on practicing and playing. I told him that I wonder if his *guilt*, and rage associated with guilt about playing, have contributed to his pain.

He hasn't told his wife that he's in psychotherapy, fearing her disapproval even though she's the one who told him about Dr. Sarno. "When she blows up, I clam up. I have to get over not being able to confront her. I'm overly concerned about how she'll react and feel," particularly about his expenditures on musical instruments, their computer, and their car. It seems to me that he has allowed his wife to take a parental role, but I don't make this observation at this point. We are working hard on helping him speak up when he needs to.

(3/8/04) Mr. A begins the session by speaking about his good qualities: extraordinary patience, empathy for people in tough situations, no prejudice, very open, and people-smart. It has been important to be receptive to his daughter, who can be so sensitive to others but not to him. Wife would say, why don't you come right out and say what's on your mind? She would say I blame her for what's not right, that I overthink things, that I've been more withdrawn and detached. Positive things his wife would say: I'm a devoted father and husband, a good wage earner, keep my sense of humor and try to have fun, I'm kind, unselfish, not afraid to go the extra mile. I've been there for her and her family.

(3/26/04) Reports that on the eve of the anniversary of his brother's death, he developed a gout attack. Although he is feeling more confident at work he still contrasts himself unfavorably with his brother: "I could never be as strong as my brother and never as athletic as my next younger brother. I had to prove to my parents that I had something." Eventually, he turned it into, "I don't care about anything…" At dinner with the family, he did a lot of daydreaming and his idolized older brother would say, "Don't you have anything to say?" I was daydreaming about excelling at something. I do that with my wife and daughter also.

(3/29/04) Eager to start the session, Mr. A tells me a dream he had after the St. Patrick's Day parade:

> I'm with a friend from high school, R. He's with me at my parents' house, showing me how to cook chicken. My older brother is hobbling on crutches. My father is not feeling well. I look at the fireplace, and R is cooking our dog. She has a regal, noble bearing. Parts of her body are cooking. I was eating this meat. I woke up with an upset stomach.

His first association is to his daughter's asking for a gerbil, and then he thinks about their dog, C. He shifts to describe his last two years in high school in a new school:

> I had come from an all-boys Catholic prep school where I had discipline problems, poor grades, and I was the class clown. I had to leave for another much bigger school. I went from class clown to nobody. In high school, my older brother threw me down the stairs but he always included me with his friends. I was 14 and he was 17.

Mr. A then emphasizes the significance of the date, March 14. His brother and grandmother died on March 14. A younger sister got married on March 14 and had two daughters on that date. His most recent gout attack was on March 14. Going further with more associations about health and family connections, he told me for the first time that his older brother had a really bad back problem. "I never felt bad about it until after he died." Mr. A still has his older brother's green jacket, the one he always wore on St. Patrick's Day. R, the friend from high school in the dream, was a blowhard: "He tells me it's chicken when it's our dog." I asked how he coped with those two awful years in high school. "I got physical symptoms and developed a self-deprecating sense of humor. In the dream, it's like the dog was sweating tears. I was always trying to 'take it.'"

(4/5/04) He starts the session by telling me that September 11, 2001 was his 50th birthday, his first important birthday. "Since then, I've lost my enthusiasm. Family security is more important than progress at work." Nevertheless, he has been working on his goal in therapy:

> I'm speaking up more with Joe. My shoulder is much better. I had a dream last night. I was in *The Sopranos*. I felt trapped, like the people in *The Sopranos*. I feel stuck in areas of my life. I did it to myself. I created my situation. I didn't speak up for myself, in the interest of getting security. [FSA: How would you want to feel, instead of trapped?] I'd be free, go out to lunch, live further out in the country but I have to get my daughter educated.

Discussion

Depicting the rhythms and textures of the clinical process with six patients who came for treatment of TMS/PPD pain, I offer the reader insight and documentation of how psychological awareness can relieve pain. Restoring links between emotions and life experiences provided significant, often striking, relief from pain for my six patients. To oversimplify, they needed to be able to say, "When that happened, I felt this." "When I think about what happened or what might happen, I feel this."

Detecting feelings, or emotions, may seem like an easy first step. I documented how difficult this first step can be by tracking in detail how I worked with Ellen and Mrs. R to help them realize that they were **not aware** of having feelings about what *I* experienced as present and past circumstances that would evoke strong feelings. The therapist's skill at being aware of their own emotions as they listen to the person in pain is essential in helping that person detect "absent" and "suppressed" emotions. In describing the interactions with Ellen and Mrs. R, I gave examples of how I used awareness of my feelings to guide me in helping them learn to detect their own feelings.

At the beginning of psychotherapy, each of my six patients had difficulty knowing what they were feeling. In fact, they had learned *not to feel* and *to suppress feelings* in order to survive challenging life circumstances: Bullying by a sibling (Ellen and Mr. A); living with a spouse who was emotionally and physically threatening (Ellen); becoming self-sufficient and learning to please others too early in childhood in order to survive "inordinate benign neglect" (Ms. T); witnessing accidents (Mrs. R) and self-harming behavior during childhood (Kate); living with the loss of a first-born child (Mrs. R); coping with multiple losses in adulthood (Kate and Ms. T); and surviving harsh parenting (Mr. L).

As the person in pain begins to detect and identify a range of feelings, for example, sadness, joy, anger, guilt, shame, and fear, they need to be able to tolerate the feelings. Feelings that have been *contained in the emotional reservoir* for decades can easily feel overwhelming, as if a volcano is erupting. I described two occasions in Ellen's therapy when she almost "blacked out" in the sessions as she started to feel rage, for the first time, at her brother and her mother. In Ellen's words, "It'll make you crazy to feel forty years of what was repressed in such a concentrated fashion."

In my first session with Mrs. R, she suddenly started to weep when she told me about never having seen her first-born son. I was concerned that she would not return for a second session because she was distressed that she was experiencing intense emotions about a traumatic ambiguous loss in early adulthood. What stunned, and heartened, both of us was that she was free of pain for days after that session. This was a dramatic example of how experiencing emotions can be followed by complete relief of pain.

Thus, a crucial part of the recovery from PPD pain related to overwhelming experiences in the past is to gradually learn to identify and tolerate feelings. Then the feelings can be used effectively in relationships in the present. I always explain to my patients that feelings help us survive. Feelings tell us if there is danger or safety: do I need to fight, flee, or freeze so that I won't be noticed until the threat has passed. Some people in pain come to treatment aware of having intense feelings but have difficulty tolerating the feelings. They may or may not be aware of the relationship between these feelings and the PPD pain. For these people, the challenges are learning to tolerate the feelings and exploring the connections between these feelings and their pain.

The six patients I write about here learned long ago to freeze, to suppress, when fighting and fleeing were not options. Unfortunately, each patient grew up in circumstances in which threat and danger, to varying degrees, were ongoing possibilities. Living in an atmosphere fraught with danger, a developing child and adolescent usually does not have the option to learn to feel and tolerate anger. In treatment for PPD pain, significant work may need to be done to learn how to use anger to assert oneself, to set "boundaries" to create safety in relationships. I illustrate how Ellen, Mrs. R, Ms. T and Mr. A learned to feel anger and set limits in relationships. Referring to the central theme in Mr. A's therapy, these patients learned how to "speak up" for themselves.

Feelings of safety, pleasure, joy, and love help us bond with others, providing support to move forward in life and handle internal and external pressures. Too often, the same people who suppressed anger and fear early in life did not feel secure bonds with the power figures around them. The six patients whose treatment I described here had survived by learning to please others in order to secure a sense of safety and self-esteem. Along with pleasing others, they learned, in varying degrees, to press themselves for performance at the highest levels in all areas. I described how this kind of self-induced pressure had contributed to considerable anger deposited into the reservoir of rage.

Ms. T discovered that she had developed perfectionist demands of herself in an attempt to be liked. Mr. L said that the therapy helped him realize that "I don't have to be in a battle with myself." Choosing not to be in a battle, choosing not to critique himself harshly, led to a relief from pain for Mr. L. Kate relied on a strong sense of responsibility and integrity to cope with the stresses in her childhood years, for example, her mother's chronic depression and multiple suicide attempts. She valued her capacity to continue to work despite years of chronic pain as an adult. Her relief from PPD pain came from realizing that she needed to recognize the feelings from childhood that she had deposited in her emotional reservoir. My question at the end of the fourth of the five focused sessions, "I wonder what little Kate has been feeling throughout these challenging times?" gave her access to feelings of grief about the loss of her mother. Initiating and completing the grieving process over the next year gave Kate relief from PPD pain.

The pathways to pain relief for these six people are offered with the hope that their experiences will be useful to people in pain, to those who have loved ones in pain, and to professionals who try to help their patients find relief from pain. These narratives, created by therapist and patient, offer stimulation for thinking about one's own history of pain and inspiration to explore the emotional circumstances in one's life that may be related to the development of pain. Only a physician can make a diagnosis of PPD pain.

CONCLUSION
Eric Sherman & Frances Sommer Anderson

When the explicit connection between disavowed affect and pain symptomatology is not systematically demonstrated to people, this dynamic remains on the fringes of their awareness. It does not become integrated as a permanent, internal resource. Consequently, intolerance of one's own anger is never identified as the direct cause of the pain, and the person is deprived of an essential tool for monitoring and controlling the pain.

If affect intolerance is not seen as the culprit, the therapeutic goals shift from cure to helping the patient cope with pain. The patient is taught how to walk, bend, lift, and avoid potentially problematic activities. This misguided shift in strategy often results in people being subjected to more useless treatments, which reinforce the individual's sense of disability and hopelessness. The search for the actual cause of the pain gets sidelined as a non-issue, or is recast as a resistance to treatment.

We are just beginning to grasp the elaborate interplay between the mind and the body, especially the way it manifests itself in the treatment situation. Most therapists endorse the notion that psychological factors influence an individual's experience of pain, both favorably and unfavorably. However, few clinicians embrace the position that musculoskeletal pain can originate from within the mind, as a means to protect an individual from unbearable emotional distress. Until the mental health and medical communities tentatively accept the psychophysiologic basis of musculoskeletal pain and other mindbody disorders, our work can neither be effectively challenged or supported. Our work with Dr. Sarno's patients represents an initial foray into the field of psychophysiologic medicine with a very specific subset of individuals suffering from chronic pain syndromes. These observations may not always apply to different clinical subgroups, or other psychological formulations of pain symptomatology and psychophysiologic disease. Nevertheless, my colleagues and I invite vigorous debate and research that may lead to more effective treatments for the widespread disability and suffering associated with incorrectly diagnosed psychophysiologic pain disorders.

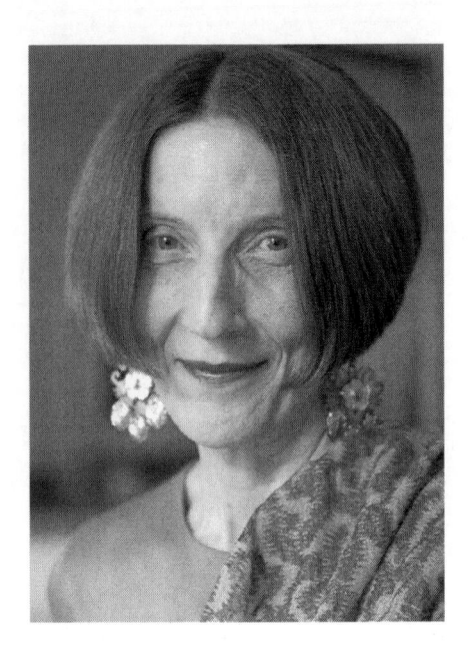

Frances Sommer Anderson, PhD, SEP, a licensed psychologist in New York State, holds a Certificate of Specialization in Psychotherapy and Psychoanalysis from New York University and a Somatic Experiencing Practitioner (SEP) certificate from the Somatic Experiencing Trauma Institute. She is in full-time private practice in New York City. Her most recent publication, *Bodies in Treatment: The Unspoken Dimension* (The Analytic Press, 2007), is an edited collection of articles at the leading edge of theoretical and clinical explorations of nonverbal communication in the psychoanalytic process. With Lewis Aron, she co-edited a pioneering book, *Relational Perspectives on the Body* (The Analytic Press, 1998), which is recognized as a major contribution on the place of the body in contemporary psychoanalytic theory. Dr. Anderson is a founding Board Member of the PPDA (Psychophysiologic Disorders Association).

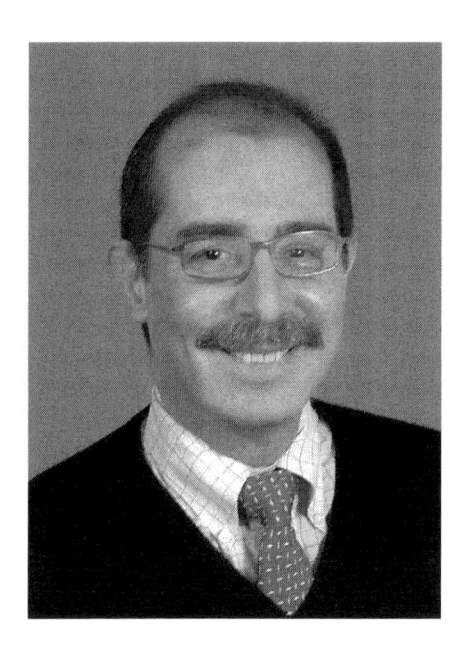

Eric Sherman, PsyD, a licensed psychologist in New York City, received a certificate of Specialization in Psychoanalysis and Psychotherapy from The New York University Postdoctoral Program in Psychotherapy and Psychoanalysis. He has a full-time private practice in New York City. Dr. Sherman is a founding Board Member of the PPDA (Psychophysiologic Disorders Association).

John E. Sarno, MD, a graduate of Columbia University College of Physicians and Surgeons, is Board Certified in Physical Medicine and Rehabilitation and Professor of Rehabilitation Medicine, New York University School of Medicine. Author of four books on pain disorders in the period 1984 to 2006, he advanced the pioneering idea that back pain and other related disorders are often psychophysiologic disorders, not due to structural abnormalities or disease processes.

For more information, please visit:
http://pathwaystopainrelief.com/

Printed in Great Britain
by Amazon.co.uk, Ltd.,
Marston Gate.